To Three and Beyond

Stories of Breastfed Children and the Mothers Who Love Them

Edited by
Janell E. Robisch

Praeclarus Press, LLC
2504 Sweetgum Lane
Amarillo, Texas 79124 USA
806-367-9950
www.PraeclarusPress.com

DISCLAIMER
The information contained in this publication is advisory only and is not intended to replace sound clinical judgment or individualized patient care. The author disclaims all warranties, whether expressed or implied, including any warranty as the quality, accuracy, safety, or suitability of this information for any particular purpose.

ISBN: 978-1-939807-16-8

Cover Design: Ken Tackett
Acquisition & Development: Kathleen Kendall-Tackett
Copy Editing: Name: Judy Torgus
Layout & Design: Cornelia Georgiana Murariu
Operations: Scott Sherwood

Table of Contents

Acknowledgments

First and foremost, I want to thank my children, A.J., Lily, and Ginny, who have taught me more about myself than perhaps anyone else, and who have given me the confidence and the privilege to love them, nurture them, and mother them through these early years.

I also thank my husband and my extended family, who supported me through my parenting journey with not much more than raised eyebrows, even when we didn't agree. I certainly can't forget all of the mothers who have contributed to this project, both in its first stages and in the later ones. Even those who just sent an email to say, *"Me, too!,"* and those whose tales did not make it into the book are important to me, as are all of the other mothers out there who are nursing or have nursed their children past our cultural norm.

Thank you.

Notes

Although only some instances have been noted at the request of individual authors, all of the authors and photographers in this book hold the rights to their own stories and photos. These should not be copied without their permission.

There are some inconsistencies in the way that each mother's name and location are listed, but this was done with purpose. They are all listed exactly how the authors wanted to list them, whether mostly anonymously or completely accurately. This allowed me to gather stories from all who wanted to share without impinging on any author's privacy.

Introduction

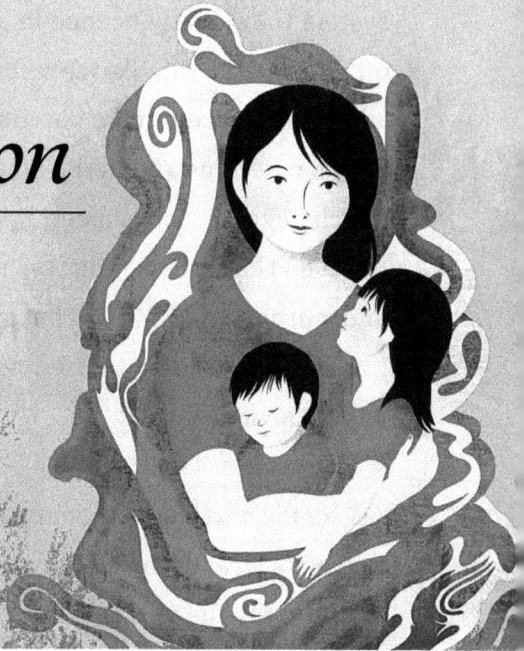

When I became pregnant for the first time in 2000, I knew that I would breastfeed. Not personally knowing anyone who had breastfed beyond a few weeks, I read as much as I could while I was pregnant and in the early days of breastfeeding to sustain and manage the nursing relationship that I now shared with my son. What I didn't know then was how long I would choose to breastfeed. I figured at least a year, especially after we got past those first few weeks and everything seemed to get easier. Nursing him made me realize how important physical closeness and attachment were, not just to him as the baby, but to me as well. It helped to foster my mothering instincts and behaviors to the point that I felt very connected to him in a way that helped me meet his needs: to help him grow and learn to the best of his potential.

When my son was 10 months old, I attended my first La Leche League (LLL) meeting and finally started to gather the support system that I badly needed in a society where breastfeeding is not often seen, despite its many benefits. It was very reassuring and even empowering to be surrounded by like-minded mothers both at LLL meetings and in the playgroup that I attended with my son, which began at those meetings. These were mothers who, like me, believed that breast milk was not only the superior way of feeding and mothering your baby, but also the natural way, the normal way. I was so inspired by this fellowship, this sisterhood, that I became an LLL Leader myself.

Over the next few years, mothering through breastfeeding continued to feel natural to me and my son. Granted, there were times when I wished that he would slow down or at least not nurse at night. He was a very demanding nurser. He insisted on it as if it were included in a Child's Bill of Rights (which perhaps it should be). I learned over time by listening to my son and by trusting my instincts that this was one of the ways that he was telling me that he still needed to nurse. He still needed that closeness and that guaranteed time with me. He still needed the nutritional and immunological benefits that come with nursing at any age. If I pulled away, he clung more. So, time passed, and as his second, third, and even fourth birthdays passed, he was still nursing.

A combination of events led me to feel more and more alone in nursing my son as he got older. First, the women in my playgroup, then nine of us, had all become very close friends. Some of the mothers got pregnant again. All of the playgroup moms that I knew continued to nurse during pregnancy, at least in the beginning. However, two children weaned on their own during pregnancy, and another was weaned by her mother as the birth of the second child grew close. Each mother followed her own instincts, and we respected one other, even when those decisions were different from our own. Then, one mother, who was nursing her 2½-year-old son, moved from our area in northern Virginia to Hawaii. Suddenly, I was the mother of the oldest nursling in our little playgroup! My son was only 2½, but the other two children in playgroup that were older than him had already weaned. A year later, we moved west from northern Virginia to the Shenandoah Valley. Our new hometown was very small, and it was very rare to see someone nursing a newborn, let alone a 3½-year-old.

I still felt that the continuation of our nursing relationship was not only natural but necessary to my son's well-being. However, I began to fear the consequences of revealing this to new friends and neighbors. Although I nursed him mostly at home now, I did attend an LLL meeting about 45 minutes away and eventually started a group in my new town. Still, getting to know others was a slow process. I took my son back to our playgroup in northern Virginia at regular intervals so we wouldn't lose our regular support network while we built up a new one.

The fear and discomfort got to me, though. It nagged at me. I looked for more venues of support. As an LLL Leader and avid reader, of course, I knew about the wonderful information in *Mothering Your Nursing Toddler* by Norma Jane Bumgarner, which I had read when my son was about 15 months old. I knew about Katherine Dettwyler's research, which suggested that the natural age of weaning was somewhere between the ages of 2.5 and 7. I was fortunate to also know several mothers who practiced child-led weaning, or at least *"very extended"* breastfeeding. However, I still felt part of a very small minority. I felt that someone needed to address the needs of mothers who were nursing children past toddlerhood, past the age of 3. Little did I know that I was far from the only closet nurser out there!

In May 2005, when my son was 4½, in an attempt to widen the base of information and support on this topic, I decided that I wanted to write about nursing beyond the age of 3. I wanted to move social thinking forward to a place where mothers would be able to listen to their own inner voice about what was right for them and their families. I wanted them to know that nursing beyond age 3 into the preschool years, and sometimes into the school years, is not only normal but can also be beneficial and surprisingly wonderful.

When I started, I did not yet know if I wanted to write an article or a book. My first attempt at the project, however, showed me that there was a definite need for the subject to be covered. I eventually heard from almost 500 women over the Internet who had nursed a child past the age of 3. Some of these women answered an extended survey for me and shared stories and photos, which were to be the basis of my book on long-term nursing.

However, as so often happens when you have young children, life got in the way while my file cabinet sat full of information and stories waiting to be shared. First, after six years of trying and one miscarriage, I finally had another baby, a daughter. Twenty-one months and one big surprise later, we welcomed our third child, another daughter, into our family. This era proved to be a very intense time for our family, as just when we were adjusting to having three kids in the house, my son's unique needs became very apparent. Less than a year after our third child was born, A.J. was diagnosed with Asperger's syndrome. I was also suffering from chronic pain that had started during my pregnancy with my third child and never seemed to stop. Those two or three years are kind of a blur for me, and I am happy to have pictures to jog my memory. Needless to say, I was so busy living and dealing with life that there was not much time for writing books.

Through almost all of this time, I was still nursing, pregnant, or both. My son eventually weaned at the age of 5. I've included his weaning story in Chapter 6. My first daughter followed in his footsteps and nursed until shortly before her fifth birthday. My younger daughter, never one to be left behind, weaned *"early"* at age 3½.

However, the thought of this book never left my mind, even after Ann Sinnot, with whom I had corresponded early on, published her book *Breastfeeding Older Children.* Although I thought that my book would complement Sinnot's rather than compete with it, something about my project just wasn't clicking for me. Then, one day in 2013, when I was paging through another book, I realized that it was all about my approach. When I had collected surveys early on, the most interesting part of them for me had been the mothers' stories. I relished reading firsthand what each mother had experienced and how each had handled various situations in the life of a breastfeeding mother. It was more than just answers to questions. It was like an LLL meeting on paper, specially designed for full-term breastfeeding mothers. From that point on, the book progressed at a rapid pace. I found a publisher with Praeclarus Press, a small press dedicated to women's health and run by Kathleen-Kendall Tackett, a well-known name in breastfeeding circles. Right away, I started a blog, a Twitter feed, and a Facebook page and published a call for stories, asking mothers to share with me—and the world—their experiences with breastfeeding beyond the third birthday.

In the months since then, I have received many stories and words of encouragement from mothers around the world. These women have shared their journeys, their photos, and their hopes and fears. They have shared everything from their decisions to continue breastfeeding into *"the beyond,"* to their stories of breastfeeding under special circumstances, to tales of how their breastfeeding journeys ended.

I hope that their stories, short and sometimes humorous quotations, photographs, and artwork will be of help to you on your journey whether you are nursing a baby, toddler, preschooler, or school-age child. Alternatively, if you are the partner, spouse, friend, or family member of a mother who is nursing full-term or just want to learn more about this unique and wonderful relationship, I applaud you for seeking out this information and hope that what you find here will be helpful to you as well.

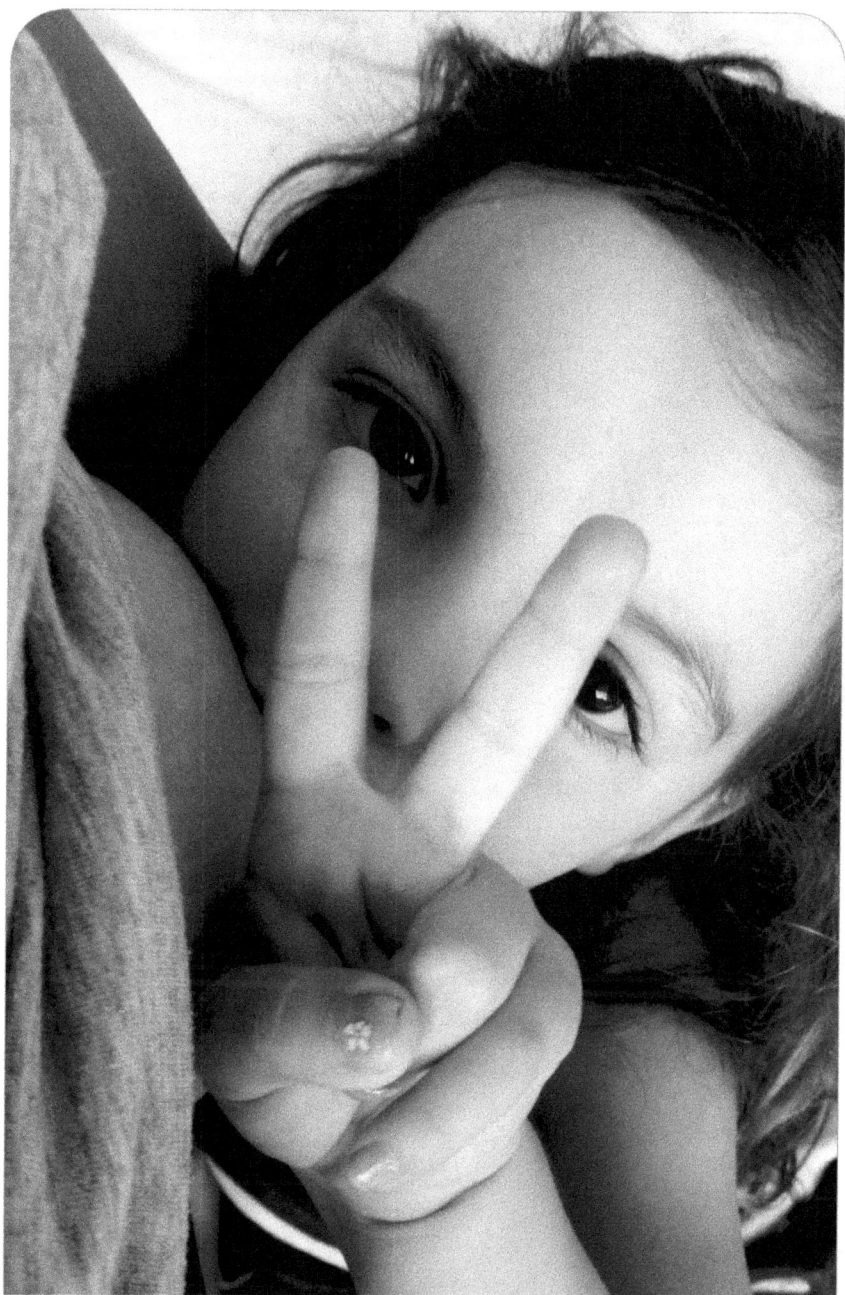

Photographed by Jasmine N. Krapf.

© 2014 Jasmine N. Krapf.

Chapter 1

How Did We Go from Three Weeks to Three Years?

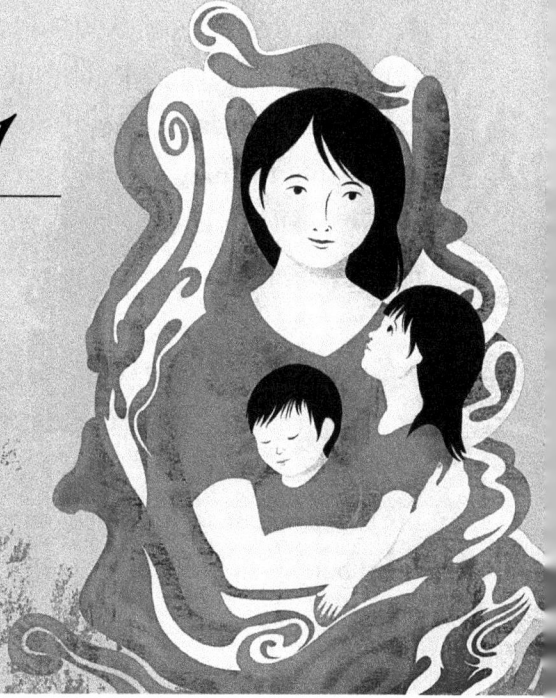

It is unlikely that the majority of women, upon first learning that they will soon be a mother, state, *"Three years. That's it. Three years is my goal for breastfeeding."* In this day and age, many mothers strive for six weeks, six months, or maybe a year. So how does this change during the course of early parenting or during the parenting of subsequent children? How do mothers and families decide that long-term nursing is the right thing—and perhaps really the normal thing—to do?

Normal or Radical?
Jessica Dee Humphreys, Canada

From religion to toilet paper roll placement, our *"normal"* develops from what we are exposed to, especially when we are young. These are the routines of daily life that we take for granted, that we don't even consider defining us because they belong to everyone we know—our families, our neighbors, our friends—but as we grow and are exposed more to the larger world, a fundamental truth reveals itself: one person's normal may be another person's radical.

I am an only child, so I didn't witness breastfeeding much growing up. The first of my girlfriends to have kids breastfed her firstborn for four years: through another pregnancy with two years of tandem nursing and yet another pregnancy. He self-weaned only when the third baby was born. Presumably, there just weren't enough boobs to go around.

This was my normal. The kids (now all enjoying their teens) were funny, healthy, loving, loud, messy, smart, and nursing.

When my son was born, I never questioned that he would breast-feed as much and as long as he liked. It was a nonissue. Like so many parenting strategies, it was mere instinct and common sense to my partner and me. We never considered bottle feeding any more than circumcision or sleep training, and we were amused to discover that we were unwittingly part of a movement called attachment parenting. Dr. William Sears's invaluable *The Baby Book* became a bible to us, not by providing information but in authorizing our gentlest and most respectful instincts toward this precious little person. Similarly, the pithy book *Happiest Baby on the Block* by Harvey Karp backed up our strong impulses to cuddle, hold, and sleep with our newborn, to rock him and wear him in a wrap or sling, to hum, sing, and shush to him—and to nurse him, like, all the time.

I had expected breastfeeding to come as naturally to me as breathing. I did not, however, anticipate the slow letdown created by my emergency C-section, the toe-curling pain of split nipples caused by the urgent sucking of a famished 10-pound baby, or the pitiful howls of hunger emitting from a newborn rapidly losing weight.

Support through Western medicine was proffered and, in my postpartum panic, was deeply appreciated. Doctors performed an emergency cesarean section after 36 hours of home labor; nurses taught awkward, but functional, breastfeeding and pumping techniques. Dr. Jack Newman's prescription nipple cream healed me overnight, and a kindly neighbor stepped in with the grateful baby's first and only bottle of formula.

When the pain and pressure finally lifted, my milk came in, rich and thick with a startlingly powerful stream. We were now able to embark on the natural and joyful journey we had hoped for. Breastfeeding became the most natural and easiest thing we did.

It was so easy, in fact, that we soon discovered it was useful as far more than just food. This free, portable, sterile, healthy snack and beverage was also a miraculous catchall of problem solvers: a sleep inducer, sleep extender, fever tamer, and air-cabin-pressure reliever; a joy maker, cuddle instigator, and guaranteed boo-boo soother. What started as de rigueur became an active (or, more accurately, a lazy) choice, as my new-mom exhaustion gave way to mother-of-an-active-toddler exhaustion, and then to I-haven't-had-a-good-night's-sleep-in-years exhaustion. Breastfeeding was easier than sleep training, bottle sterilizing, and most of all, weaning.

As the months turned to years, breastfeeding resources continued to support us. The *fin de millennium* world that set the stage for our parenting years saw the publication of *The Baby Book*; the rise of the attachment parenting movement; the United Nations' Innocenti Declaration on the Protection, Promotion, and Support of Breast-feeding; the World Health Organization's Global Strategy for Infant and Young Child Feeding; and the start of La Leche League online. Long-term breastfeeding had become a highly respected parenting technique, not only in developing countries, but here in North America, where the former U.S. Surgeon General Antonia Novello made the beautiful assertion that it is a lucky baby who nurses to age 2.

Even our pediatrician (a ruthless, old-school, cry-it-out-style doctor whom we quickly abandoned for our sweet family general practitioner) told me that she would give me until the baby turned 2 before she'd begin berating me for nursing. Other moms who weaned early were often a little wistful when they saw us, and I reveled in the warmth of indulgent smiles from strangers that we would receive.

Nursing toddlers had staunch support, and we breastfed cheerfully and freely for over two years. However, that two-year mark soon came and went. The mothers around us were weaning quickly and furiously, fed up with feeding and the accompanying sleeplessness, and support from experts was drying up fast.

It was hard for a while, not having that coterie of like-minded mommies and expert support anymore. I could see that we had slipped from normal to radical, but the ease and joy that we continued to experience from nursing kept me confident in the fact that it was still perfectly natural, even if it was not the norm. Every young child in our neighborhood still indulged (or desired to indulge) the urge to suckle. All the 4- and 5-year-olds on our block still drank from baby bottles; sucked soothers, thumbs, and backpack straps; or simply verbally lamented the loss of the breast.

A friend in the throes of a divorce took her 8-year-old to a child psychologist to get advice and was told that it was not unnatural for a child to unconsciously seek out its mother's nipple for comfort well into the tweens.

To turn to the animal kingdom for a less controversial perspective, the only other land mammal that shares our longevity, the elephant, nurses to upwards of five years. At 4½, mamma's milk is still my son's favorite thing in the world. Not only is it *"the most delicious,"* but he associates it with the safest, warmest, cuddliest, most loving experience of his life. I do ask him from time to time when he thinks that he can have *"no more milk."* His reactions range from incredulity to heartbreak and usually end in sobs that can be soothed only at the breast. However, when he's in the mood to talk, he explains, *"I still have a little baby in me,"* and that baby needs milk.

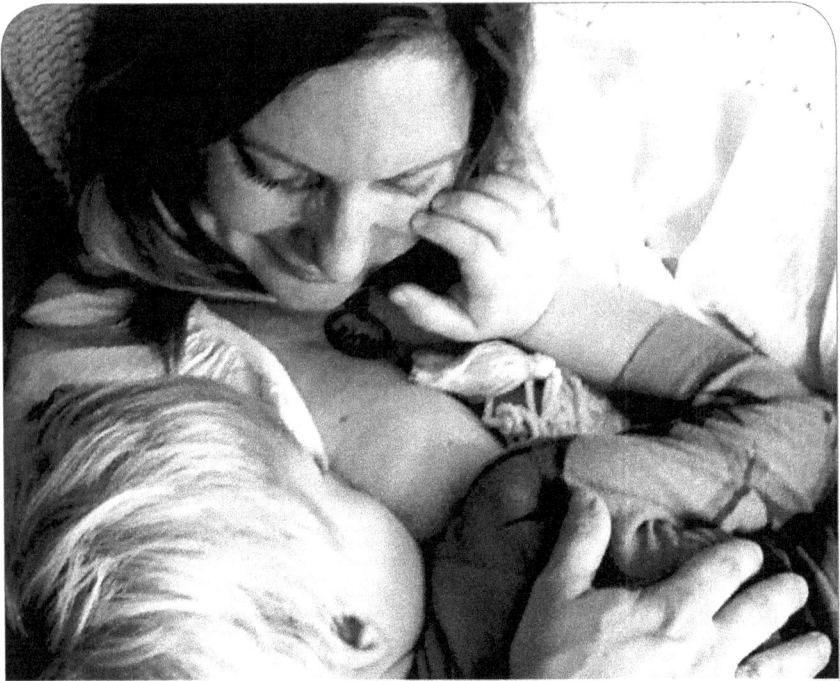

This tender touch on the cheek from Jessica's nursling reminds her that among all of its other benefits, nursing teaches nurturing.

©2013 Jessica Dee Humphreys.

Is it normal to indulge a natural, healthy instinct? Of course! Is it also normal to follow the overt conventions of our larger society? Definitely! Is there a single universally accepted norm on this or any topic? There is not.

When I consider whether long-term nursing was a mistake, I laugh to myself: we all parent differently, with greater and lesser successes, and if this is the worst parenting mistake that I make, this is some lucky kid! I know that the time is coming when he will stop, and until then, we will proceed mindfully, lovingly, and respectfully both of the baby that is still in him and the man that he will become.

Milkies Make Everything Better

Liandra Losardo, Austin, Texas

When I began breastfeeding, I had no time frame in mind. I literally took it one day at a time. Unfortunately, I didn't start doing adequate research on breastfeeding until I was in my third trimester, but once I started, I couldn't stop. I was on the La Leche League website multiple times a day and read its wonderful book, *The Womanly Art of Breastfeeding.* Between those two valuable resources, I knew breastfeeding was the way to go. It just made sense to me.

The first few months were the hardest. I was nursing on demand and at home by myself. Some days were easy, and some were downright frustrating, but I kept going. Despite the struggles, I had no real reason to stop breastfeeding. I knew that it was just my emotions getting in the way of what I knew was best. By most standards, I probably had a great start. I got mastitis only twice, and my son wasn't awake for long stretches at night, so I held onto that.

On one particular day, I had been nursing on the couch for pretty much the whole day. My husband walked in from work, and when he looked at me, I immediately began to cry. I needed a break. I felt like this stage was never going to end. This was my life, and it felt so lonely. That day, I came close to reaching for one of the many cans of formula that had been given to us—formula that, before I had learned about the magic of breastfeeding, I had planned on using—but I didn't because, if I had, I knew that doing so would only get easier. For me, it was just an easy way out, and my son deserved better than that. He deserved a mother that would stay strong and determined.

At 15 months, my son got his first fever. At that age, many kids have already had a few colds or ear infections. I knew that it was because of breast milk that my son's immune system was strong. Before I knew it, I was nursing a 2½-year-old. At this point, I wasn't going to stop breastfeeding as long as my son was happy to continue, and he was! By this time, he had gotten roseola, his first big illness. Knowing that I could comfort and nourish him all at once made it easier on all of us. I'll admit that sometimes I put too much pressure on breast milk. I had it in my head that all of this liquid gold would keep him from ever getting sick. Of course, that wasn't realistic, but what it did do was make those colds less frequent and less intense.

By the time he was 3, my son was still nursing. I began to wonder if he was ever going to wean. Long gone were the days of hour-long nursing sessions, but he was still very much a lover of his *"milkies."* My husband would tell him that he would have to stop drinking the milkies soon. He was joking, but I think that he may have meant it a little because, every now and then, I would get the *"So, when do you think you're gonna stop breastfeeding him?"* question. At this point, I was on the fence. Part of me felt that three years of breastfeeding was an amazing feat and that it would be a good time to wean him. The other part of me got sad at the thought of never getting that bonding again. I wasn't ready for this wonderful stage in my life to be over. I never would have thought I would become a supporter of child-led weaning, but how could I take away something that made my little boy so happy? I couldn't. I didn't.

A few months before his fourth birthday, he was diagnosed with RSV (respiratory syncytial virus). It was the worst that I had ever seen him. He slept most of the day, and when he was awake, he was crying. The doctor said it was something that had to run its course. I couldn't do anything to make him feel better except nurse him.

In March 2013, I was officially nursing a 4-year-old. What?! This had started to become surreal. Most women that I knew who had breastfed their toddlers were now telling their weaning stories. Not me. Although our nursing relationship had turned into two or three sessions at night and flybys during the day, I couldn't say he was weaned. As I write this, my son is 4½ years old and still gets his milkies. Sometimes, he will go all day without it (if he's preoccupied enough), but he still looks for it at night.

So, how did we get here? How did we go from day 1 to year 4? Time, patience, knowledge, support, and determination are how we got here. Taking it one day at a time and not setting limits are how we got here. The knowledge and true belief in my heart that what I was doing was the best thing for my son is how we got here. The support of La Leche League, my family, and my husband is how we got here. I had to prove to myself, the woman who usually gives up when things get too hard, that I could do it. I have never wanted to be more successful at anything in my life, and I would do it again in a heartbeat. My son will tell you *"milkies are for babies and big boys, too, and they make everything better."* I couldn't agree more.

It Seems Weird, and It Makes Me Uncomfortable[1]
Christine McCann, Cary, North Carolina

I never thought I would nurse a baby past age 1. My mother nursed me and said it was wonderful, but she had to stop only a few days after I was born because of a medication she needed. She always said that she regretted not being able to nurse me past the first week, but it was clear that she had never envisioned nursing a toddler!

We knew one mother who had nursed her youngest child past the age of 3, and she was considered very odd for doing so. Other than that, I wasn't really exposed to breastfeeding until I was in college and my aunt had a baby, so I had no idea what nursing was like, how long babies did it, or what the benefits were.

Years later, when I decided to have a baby, I thought that I would nurse, but I would stop once the baby got teeth. This is perhaps understandable for someone who didn't know how young babies are when they get teeth or how nursing mechanics really work. Luckily, I'm a compulsive researcher, and while investigating everything about pregnancy and birth, I learned that nursing until 12 months was recommended. So, I planned to nurse my baby and thought I would do so for a year.

Then my daughter Chloe was born, the day before I was scheduled to take a breastfeeding class at the birthing center. I nursed her in the first hour after she was born and thought that I was doing okay, but a few days later, I was in terrible pain with open wounds on my

---

1   The original version of this story appeared as a *Skeptical Mothering* blog post and can be found at http://skepticalmothering.com/?s=four

nipples. It took several months to figure out and fix all the problems: tongue tie, shallow latch, forceful letdown, oversupply, and a yeast infection. Perhaps if I'd taken that breastfeeding class before giving birth, it would have helped. As it was, I got a quick course from the school of hard knocks. For months, nursing was painful, frustrating, and confusing.

However, I hung in there because I had decided that breastfeeding was very important to me, and I felt that if I could just get through the difficulties, it would be worth it. Gradually, I healed, and we both learned to nurse better. By the time my daughter was 5 months old, nursing was a good part of our life. It was a moment to sit down and rest, to set aside all the other cares for a few minutes. It was an opportunity to cuddle and dote on my baby.

As she grew, it became more and more of a parenting tool. In addition to providing the nutrition and hydration that she needed, nursing offered soothing, reassurance, and a gateway to sleep.

Before I knew it, my baby was turning 1, yet she was still a baby. It seemed silly to try to make her stop at that point. How could nursing be recommended one day but totally useless the next? On her birthday, she wasn't a year older; she was a day older. I just didn't see the sense in stopping right then. Plus, I have to say that there was a certain determination on my part after we got through all those difficulties. I didn't want to give up so soon after it had finally started working! So, we kept going, and nursing continued to be useful: quelling tantrums, making nap time peaceful, and serving as a nutritional safety net.

Ironically, about a month after her first birthday, Chloe had a nursing strike. I was beside myself when my *"old reliable"* was no longer available. I fretted because she was sick and I couldn't give her extra fluids and nutrition by nursing. I hated that she was in pain from a cold and a subsiding ear infection and her typical way of getting comfort was suddenly not an option. I felt like a bond between us had been abruptly severed—I was prepared for her to wean herself over time but not to have our nursing relationship snatched away unexpectedly and all at once. Luckily, with patience and persistence, I helped her get back to nursing within a few days, and it was clear she wasn't ready to stop—she just couldn't stand to nurse when her ears hurt and her nose was stuffed up! I'm glad I didn't just give up at that point.

By the time Chloe turned 2, I was a member of La Leche League, and I had a community where nursing children until they are ready to stop was perfectly normal. I really couldn't see a positive reason to make her wean when she showed no inclination to stop breastfeeding. Nursing was still a useful parenting tool, and it was something my daughter enjoyed and benefited from.

On the other side of the scale, the arguments for weaning were weak to say the least. The predominant argument people have against continued nursing boils down to *"It seems weird, and it makes me uncomfortable."* My husband had the least dumb reservation about my nursing a 2-year-old. He said, *"If it were me, it would drive me nuts to have such a big kid lying in my lap so often."* Since it didn't bother me, and other people's argument of *"Ew!"* was unconvincing to me, we kept going.

Chloe turned 4 years old shortly after I became pregnant with Claire. Around that time, it started to really hurt me when she nursed. Aha!—a good reason to wean to balance against the arguments for continuing to nurse. Given her age, I felt comfortable telling her that nursing was hurting me and that I needed to stop. Of course, by that time she had been *"weaning"* for years, so she only nursed at bedtime by the time I decided to stop. It was relatively easy to substitute a sippy cup of water and lots of cuddling, and we were done.

Of course, with my second child, it seemed perfectly natural from the beginning that I would nurse her for years. As time went by and she turned 4 herself, I thought about it and decided that I would feel uncomfortable nursing a 5-year-old. That was just my personal, arbitrary, gut-feeling limit. (For the record, I would never tell any mother that she should nurse beyond her own emotional comfort zone, be that three months or three years.) I started subtly discouraging nursing. She had naturally pared down to nursing just at bedtime long before her fourth birthday, and shortly after turning 4, she began forgetting on occasion or wanting only one side. Finally, for various reasons, we moved the girls into the same bedroom, and unexpectedly, this caused Claire to totally wean. The shakeup in her bedtime routine, along with the security of having her sister nearby, seemed to extinguish her need for that last nighttime connection with mom.

People might be shocked to learn that my kids are both independent and socially adept. Both of them were eager and excited to hop on the school bus and spend all day at kindergarten, and they didn't spare a look back at me as they went off. They make friends easily and feel confident and secure enough to explore and go do their own thing. They're normal kids and maybe even more independent than average. People might also be surprised that Chloe has no memory of nursing. Claire has some vague memories, but I wouldn't be surprised if they fade as well.

Ultimately, I feel that nursing was just like cuddling or hugging my babies. We did it all the time at first; they needed it for their health and well-being as well as their emotional comfort. As they grew, our relationship changed. Our physical connections gradually attenuated in a healthy and natural way. My 10-year-old never announced that she was done with sitting on my lap; she simply evolved over time so that now she connects with a brief hug or by playing a game or reading with me rather than snuggling up, and so it was with nursing. They both expressed less and less need for it until it became a last touchstone before sleep, and finally, it was no longer needed. It was a wonderful journey, and I'm glad I let it continue. Every mother should feel comfortable continuing for as long as it feels right to her and her child, whether that's for four months or for four years.

Natural, Not Forced
Brandy J. Hansen, IBCLC, Normal, Illinois[2]

I don't know why it happened that my younger daughter, Ripley, nursed for so long, just that it did. There wasn't a plan to go for a certain period of time, although deep inside I hoped that it would carry into her toddlerhood—at least long enough for her to have memories of it. I guess that kind of goes back to my experience nursing my older daughter, Max. I really enjoyed it the first time around and was really looking forward to doing it again. Especially because I was a working mom, I considered nursing to be kind of a consolation prize for me having to go to work and missing the first steps, first words, etc. Nursing was a really important way for me to stay connected.

When Max weaned, it was rather abruptly at 20 months, and I have to admit, I took it really hard. I took it almost personally, and it caused more of an emotional upheaval than I had thought it would. Given that her weaning felt so harsh to me, I couldn't fathom what a little one must go through when a mom stops cold turkey—it must be even more devastating for the child! It was, in part, because of that first, sudden end to nursing that I hoped that the next time around would be better paced; maybe the kiddo would give me time to wean myself from her or at least give me some warning before deciding she didn't need me anymore.

As it turned out, my fears about a premature rejection were unrealized, and the second time around was much easier—and even more amazing.

2   IBCLC stands for International Board Certified Lactation Consultant.

The other big part of extended nursing for us was a mutual need after the stress of the pregnancy and the need for change in our family life. After having a completely uneventful and healthy first run with my older daughter, my second pregnancy was marked by premature labor at 25 weeks.

After two more bouts of labor, a helicopter ride, a month of bed rest, and shots in my rear for close to three months, it was only natural that we savored the state of being a healthy mother and child. I wanted to be close and take her in every moment that I could after her birth, and she was more than happy to oblige. I was thankful that she was here, that she was alive. The closeness and being able to do something so unique as nursing was something I desperately needed at that time in my life—as a mother, a woman lacking confidence in my body and myself—and nursing built us both up. During every morning snuggle, every nighttime nursing, and each fuss and fight that was calmed at the breast, I could feel a sort of instinctive strength growing in myself and in Ripley.

Nursing was something that calmed her as she grew, and it was part of our relationship that we both just really enjoyed and looked forward to. There was something very peaceful about having her next to me. It wasn't as easy to maintain socially as she got older; there was a lot of pressure from family and friends to wean her, and I heard, *"She's old enough!"* more times than I can count. It was hard to explain to someone who hadn't been there that my daughter didn't just magically stop needing me just because she had hit this predetermined age when nursing in our society *"should"* have stopped. Kids—hell, people—don't work that way. We continue to need contact and affection for our entire lives. I didn't stop finding comfort in her at a year, and she didn't stop coming to me at 2. At a little over 3 years old, she decided that she was confident enough to go out into the world without *"bub,"* and by that point, she was able to make that decision for herself rather than having someone else force it upon her.

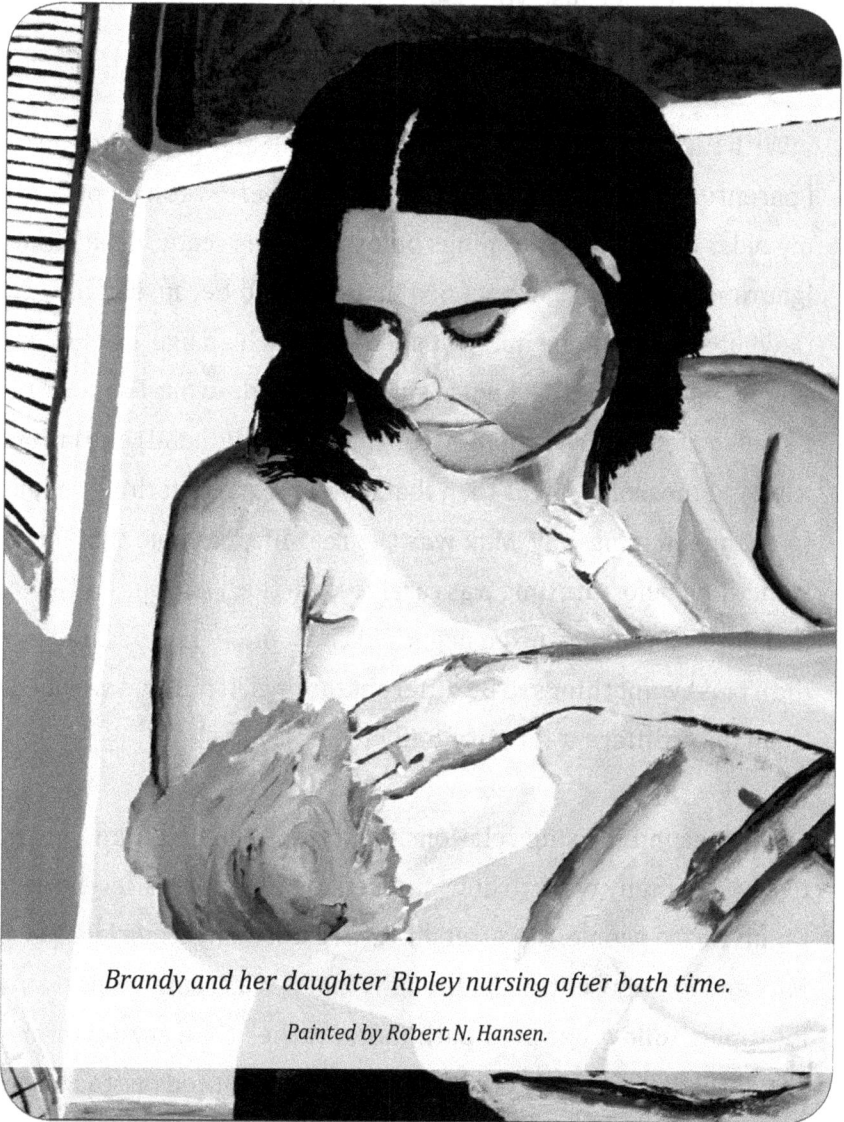

Brandy and her daughter Ripley nursing after bath time.

Painted by Robert N. Hansen.

Some people would say, *"How does a 3-year-old decide anything? You're the parent; you make the decisions,"* but that's not necessarily true, nor should it be. It's a relationship where you have to impose limits, yes, but you also have to listen to the needs of the other person. We're parents, not dictators. It's like potty training too early; you make yourself crazy trying to make your kids do something they're not ready for because you're sick of changing diapers, but if they aren't ready, it's not going to happen without disaster.

With Ripley, part of it really had to do with big changes in the way I parented once she came along. I feel like there was a lot of forcing my older daughter to do things before she was ready, mostly out of ignorance of what to expect of a little kid and because of listening to what she should be doing at such-and-such an age, but I started seeing the effects of that kind of authoritarian do-what-I-say-because-I-said-so mentality (remnants from my own childhood) on Max once Ripley came along. It was then that I understood that things needed to change in a big way. Max was the real-life example that forcing something before its time was rarely worth the headache and always had unintended (and often negative) consequences. I decided that I didn't just want things to be different for myself but that we needed them to be different for our family to survive.

This second nursing relationship softened me a bit and opened my eyes in many ways to how different people have different needs. Children are people, too, after all. As a result of my experiences with Max and my new outlook, I thought that it was really important to let Ripley follow her own path more, rather than trying to make her do what she clearly wasn't ready to do. I wanted her to have the same choice my older daughter had: to wean when she was ready (one of the few things I didn't force with her). Even with shadows of fighting and hurt feelings between my husband and me lurking in the background, she was still able to come to it naturally, without being forced, and that gives me a lot of peace.

The last time she nursed was when she was 3 years 2 months old.

Read more of Brandy's story in Chapter 4, where she elaborates on her relationship with her husband and how it affected her nursing relationship with Ripley.

We Will Not Stop Today
Marti, United Kingdom

I was born in the 1970s in Eastern Europe. Unlike Western mothers, Easterners were expected to breastfeed, even if the practices around birth were anything but helpful for breastfeeding initiation. It didn't work out for my mum, so I was bottle-fed. Feeding in public (breast or bottle) was just not done in those days. Young babies were taken out for walks in the pram, and that was it. They had their milk at home.

I was in my 20s when I first saw a baby breastfeed. It seemed so easy that I decided I would give it a try. When I got pregnant, I went to antenatal classes and learned something about breastfeeding, too, but I didn't know much, nor did I realize how much was there to know.

I didn't feel particularly passionate about the subject. I was too focused on the birth, and the birth didn't go the way I had planned. I did everything *"right"* to have a natural birth, and yet I ended up with a C-section. I thought that if the birth went well, everything else would go well too, and if the birth didn't go well, all would be doomed. As I was recovering from the surgery, I tried putting my daughter to the breast, not having much hope that she would feed, but she did!

I never had a plan for how long to breastfeed. I was due back to work nine months after her birth, and I thought that we'd be done by then. The beginning was hard. I had literally every problem in the book. It was agony, yet my daughter was gaining weight fine, so

I soldiered on. Every day, I considered giving up. I dreaded every feed. At one point, I had to rub ice cubes on my nipples to numb them before each feed, they hurt so much. I was in pain between feeds too. More and more people suggested that I give up, but the more I heard *"happy mummy = happy baby"* (which implied that I should stop breastfeeding and put my own needs first instead of my baby's), the more determined I became to continue.

When my mother mentioned that she discussed my problems with a colleague of hers and that said colleague was bewildered as to *"why didn't they [doctors] just give me a jab to dry up my milk,"* I was outraged: How dare they?! How dare my mother discuss this very personal issue with a colleague behind my back? How dare they suggest that some doctor should decide whether or not I breastfeed my child? I think in a way that I was trying to prove to my mum that I was not a worse mother than she'd been. I may not have been able to birth my daughter, I may not be a perfect mum, my baby may not be a textbook baby, but I could breastfeed.

After some two months, things fell into place. I gradually started to enjoy breastfeeding. Still, I didn't really plan how long I should continue. I remember when I first saw a breastfeeding toddler; I thought that it was just wrong. Surely, toddlers didn't need it?

My daughter started having solid foods at around 6 months of age. I was very enthusiastic about baby-led weaning. I was encouraged by the stories of babies having a great appetite for a variety of healthy foods. I thought that it would be easy to gradually replace breast milk with cow's milk as a drink. However, my daughter had little interest in solid food. She lived mostly on my milk. When she first tried cheese, she had a severe allergic reaction to it. Later, she also reacted to formula; she had tolerated it fine before the cheese episode. She was seen by a specialist doctor and diagnosed with a severe allergy to milk, eggs, and nuts. They were scary times.

At that point, I decided that I would continue breastfeeding her after I returned to work. I just thought that soy formula was a poor substitute. Still, she had that in daycare, and when we were out and about, I stopped feeding her in public. However, when we were at home, she had breast milk. The doctors reassured me that she would grow out of her milk allergy soon, so I thought that I could breastfeed her until then.

There were many times that I wanted to stop, and there were many different reasons. However, she just wasn't ready, and she was still allergic to animal milk. She asked for my milk every day, though gradually we cut down to evening and morning only. If she could not have milk, she looked so sad that it broke my heart.

She is 5 now. She still has breast milk several times a week. Few people know. Children get taken by social services for no sound reason in this country, and, sadly, many people would see breast-feeding an older child as abusive. I don't know when she will wean. I try to make it clear to her that it's her choice; she can have my milk if she wants it, but she doesn't have to have it if she doesn't want it.

When she was 3, her brother was born. Even having breastfed an older child, I wasn't sure I would feed my son *"full term."* I thought that if he didn't have allergies, he would move on to cow's milk when he was 1. He didn't have allergies, but when he turned 1, he was living mostly on my milk.

This time around, I am not too stressed about pushing solids. I try to limit his daytime feeds. I try not to feed him in public, but I do sometimes and don't give a hoot what people think. I have this evil look for such occasions, so I've never had anyone approach me with any comments.

I don't know what the future will bring. I'm not much of a planner. I just take every day as it comes. I remember that when my daughter was a tiny baby and I was considering giving up, someone told me that I don't have to decide now when I would stop breastfeeding. I could simply decide that I was not going to stop today, and for the last 2000 days, I've been making the same decision.

Read more of Marti's story in Chapter 3, where she talks about balancing her desire to have more children with the immediate needs of her firstborn.

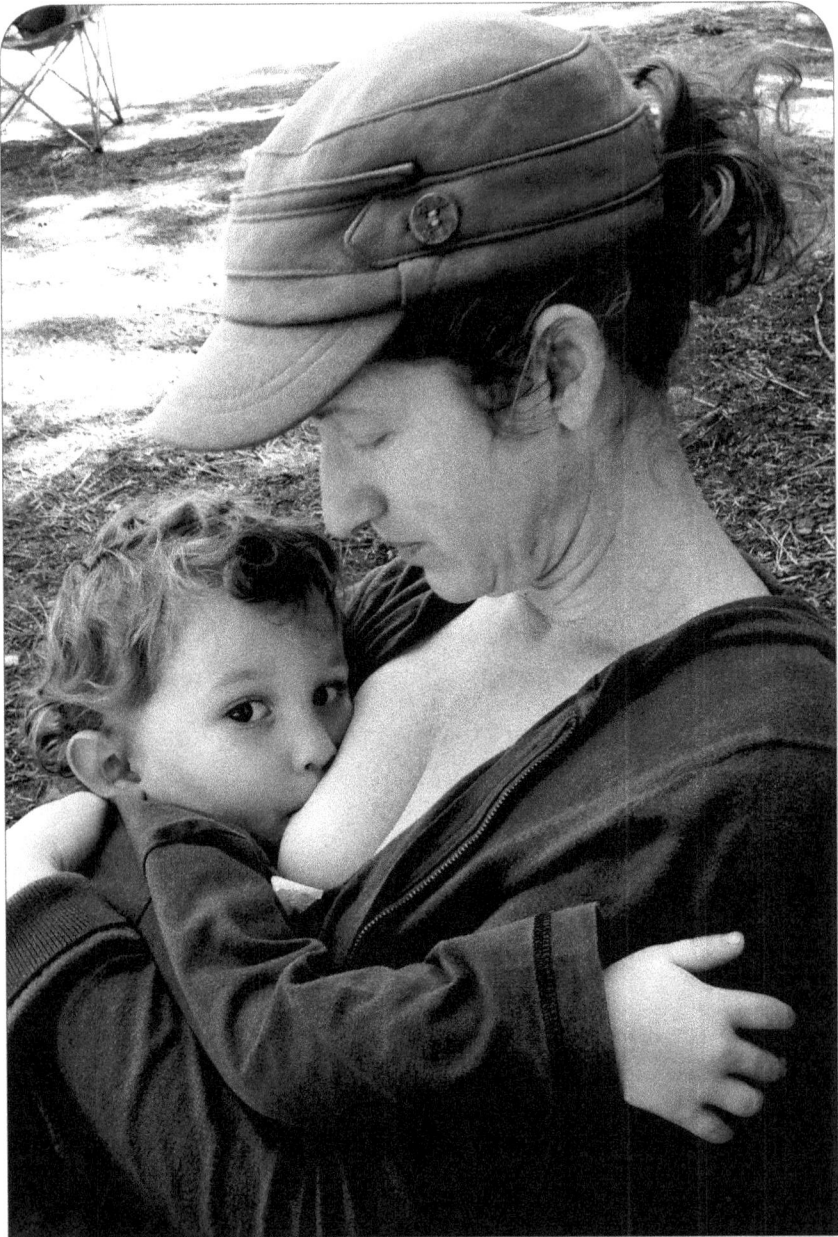

Dr. Jennie Cato, OB/GYN, and her son Braeden nursing on their annual family camping trip to the Sierra Mountains in California shortly after his third birthday. Photographed by Nathan M. Swift.

The Fourth Time is the Charm

Sharon Spink, Sherburn in Elmet, North Yorkshire, England[3]

I have four children, and all of them were breastfed at some point but for various lengths of time. My first, Kevin, who was born in 1987, was breastfed for only two weeks. Of course, I do feel guilty about this, even after 26 years, but I was very young, breastfeeding wasn't encouraged, and I had a huge lack of confidence, information, and support.

I remember happily letting him go off to the nursery in the hospital so I could have a rest. Bottles of formula were readily available on the wards. He was a large baby at 8 pounds 10 ounces, so I was convinced that I couldn't fill him and happily topped him up with formula while we were in the hospital.

My second child, Sarah, who was born in 1990, managed to feed for a little longer, but we still made it to only four weeks. Again, I think this was due to a lack of information and support; plus, I still didn't feel comfortable feeding in front of people, especially male relatives. Breastfeeding still wasn't encouraged, and formula was very much pushed by health professionals at the first sign of any problems.

She was a small baby at birth, weighing just 5 pounds 10 ounces, and so we were made aware of how much weight she wasn't gaining in comparison with the growth charts in her baby record book. So, once again, we very quickly switched her to formula.

---

3   Sharon is the owner of Booby & The Beads (https://www.facebook.com/BoobyandtheBeads). She makes jewelry for breastfeeding moms and offers breastfeeding peer support.

Some 16 years later in 2006, I had baby number three, my daughter Isabel. I had learned so much more, had loads more confidence in myself, and was determined to breastfeed.

We got off to a flying start, despite her birth being my third cesarean section. She fed beautifully within the hour, and I thought that I'd finally gotten the hang of breastfeeding. Things were going great, despite the usual sore nipples, sleepless nights, and cluster feeding, or so I thought. I used to get her weighed regularly, but when she was about 4 months old, our health visitors picked up on her weight and noticed that one week she would gain weight only to lose it again the following week. Therefore, she never gained any real weight. Their *"wonderful advice"* was to top her off with formula. Thanks so much for that amazing support!

Giving her that first bottle of formula absolutely broke my heart (and still does). I cried in the pharmacy having to buy it (I only bought a ready-made carton because I was still in denial that I was having to formula-feed), and I cried all the way through that first bottle. We managed to carry on the mixed feedings for another two months until one day she just refused to feed, and I took that as my cue to stop feeding. Maybe it was a nursing strike, and with support, maybe I could have carried on feeding her for longer, but I don't like to dwell on that memory because it hurts too much.

When Isabel was 3, along came baby number four, my daughter Charlotte, and I was adamant that I would breastfeed. She was another C-section baby, and as soon as she was born, I was talking about skin-to-skin contact. I was told to wait until I was in recovery, but the operating team was taking ages to stitch me back up and clean me up. I was panicking that it would be too late and that she wouldn't feed properly. I completely forgot to ask if she could have skin-to-skin contact with her daddy. Anyway, after what felt like ages, we finally got to recovery, and we had our lovely skin-to-skin time and her first feed.

I had a few problems with sore nipples again, but Lansinoh cream and breast milk soon sorted them out. Her growth spurts were a nightmare. Sometimes, I sat on the sofa for 12 to 15 hours at a time. Luckily, they all happened on a weekend when my husband was around to look after Isabel.

As far as I was concerned, I had failed to breastfeed three times, and so this time I was going to feed Charlotte for as long as possible. I set myself small goals: six weeks, six months, 12 months, and two years, but I knew deep down that if I could get past the initial six months, we definitely weren't looking back or thinking about stopping. I never knew then that I would be breastfeeding a school-aged child, and although I had hoped to reach the World Health Organization's recommended two years and beyond, I hadn't really visualized that in my head. We just went on from day to day, month to month, and year to year, and before I knew it, two years had come and gone.

I have done so much since she was born: started a new business, completed Breastfeeding Peer Supporter Training through my local Children's Centre, completed the Association of Breastfeeding Mothers' Mother Supporter Training, arranged a breastfeeding flash mob in Leeds, appeared on national television (ITV's This Morning in May 2012) about breastfeeding an older child, and started Breast-feeding Counsellor training, again with the Association of Breast-feeding Mothers. I love supporting other mums on their breastfeeding journeys too, and I volunteer at two local breastfeeding cafes. It's so rewarding to see mums overcoming their own problems and to know that I have given them the skills, support, and information they need to continue their own breastfeeding journeys.

Charlotte is 4 now, and I don't know how much longer she is going to want to feed. Until recently, she still had a feed during the night on most nights; she just came into our bed. Now, occasionally at bed time, she'll want a feed and always wants *"mummy milk"* if she's hurt or upset. She is showing no sign of stopping, though, and I'm more than happy for her to continue as long as she wants to.

My family has been very supportive of me breastfeeding, although I suspect hubby would like to have more room in the bed each night. I have had comments about when will I be stopping, and I just tell people it's up to Charlotte. She started full-time school in September 2013, and this hasn't affected her breastfeeding at all. We have a lovely breastfeeding relationship, and I will definitely miss it when she eventually decides it's time to stop.

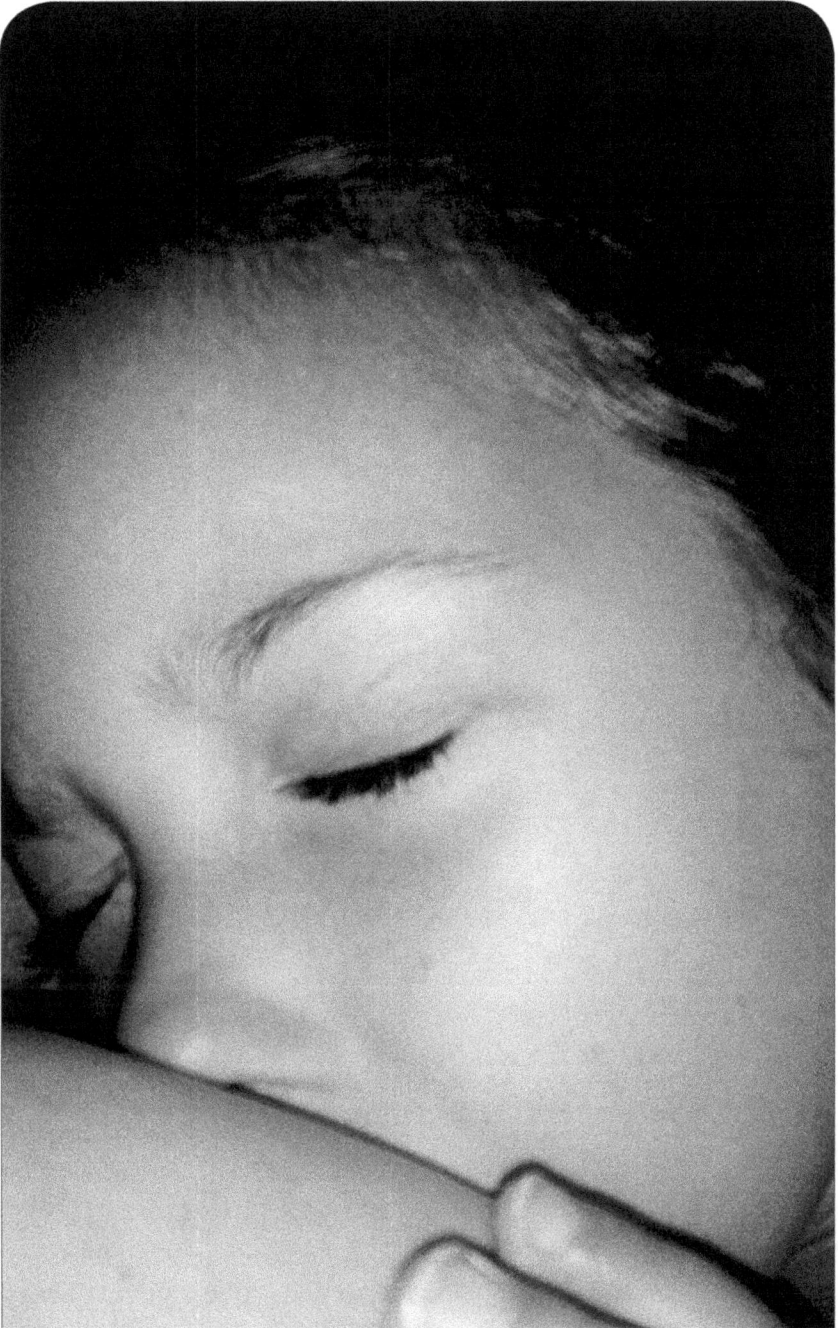

Charlotte says that this is the best way to say night, night.

Chapter 2

Advantages and Moments of Joy

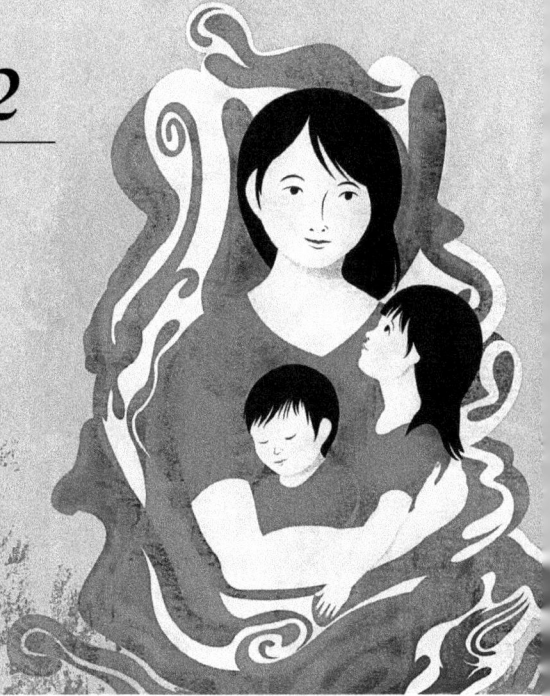

M others have many a tale to tell when it comes to breastfeeding the *"older child."* Some are not pretty. They can be filled with 3-year-olds demanding to nurse every 5 minutes, and the pain that comes from a lazy nighttime latch suddenly clamping shut. However, if it weren't for all of the advantages and moments of joy, not many of us would have ever traveled this far down the road. We all experience things a little differently, but here are some things to brighten your journey or just to make you smile.

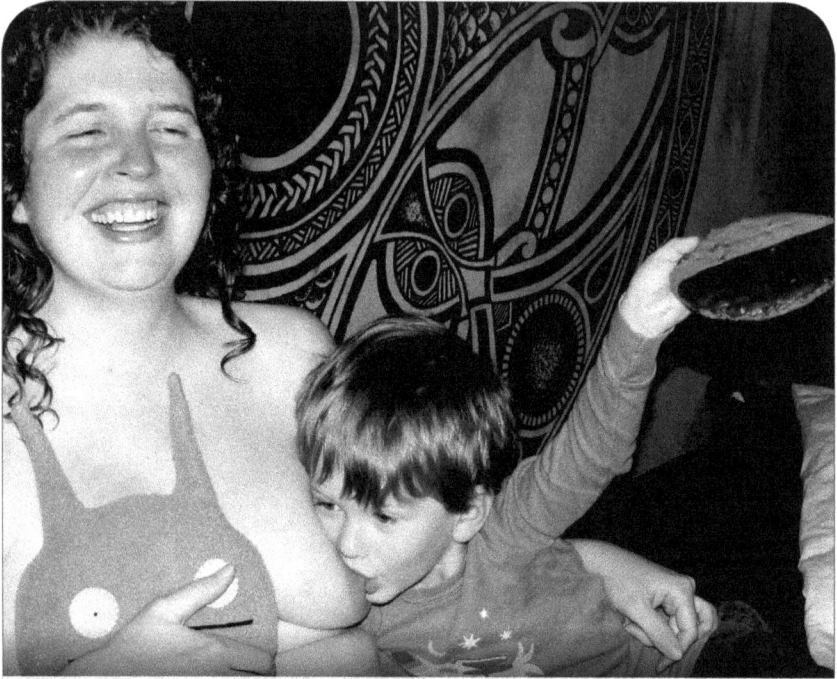

Photograph staged in response to an Oreos ad. This is a cookie for a preschooler. Pauline Osborne and son, Redmond, Washington.

Healthy, Safe, and Close to My Heart
Olivia Hinebaugh, Burke, Virginia

Any parent or caregiver of preschoolers knows that one of the joys of having them is watching them express themselves. The things that they say and do give us such a wonderful window into their world. My memories of being 3 are vague at best. I don't remember what it was like to see the world from down there, to learn such big things every day, or to rely on my parents for everything. I love hearing all about my son's life as he sees it. A great thing about nursing a 3-year-old is that he can tell you why he nurses.

It's obvious when they're babies. They nurse to eat. They nurse to be healthy. They nurse to feel safe. They nurse to be close to mom's heart.

For the questioning public at large, it's not obvious why a kid who eats real food, runs around, and dresses himself would nurse. I know why I still nurse my son: because weaning him has never seemed like the easy choice. I admit it: I still nurse him in part because it's easy. If he's having a hard day, nursing makes everything all right. It's a magic reset button. If he's hurt, nursing makes him forget until it stops hurting. If he doesn't want to lie down to go to sleep, nursing calms him, and he curls up with me easily, not fighting it. Any mom with such a powerful antidote in her toolkit would be mad not to use it!

However, nursing is only half about the mom. I wanted to know what my son, Callum, thought about nursing. He's a chatty guy and hardly needs any prompting on this subject—he feels very passionate about it. His first word, before *"Mama"* even, was *"nun,"* his word for nursing. Eventually it turned into *"wanna nun"* and *"nun peas,"* and when he became even more articulate in his third year, it was, *"Please, can I nurse?"* He always smiles and giggles happily when he asks this. Now, because everything is a *"why"* or a *"because,"* he asks, *"Please, can I nurse because I want to/because it's my favorite/because...."*

When I got pregnant with his little sister, I read up on tandem nursing. It was clear to me that he had no intention of stopping. In my research, I discovered that nature has a way of weaning children when their moms are pregnant.

I started asking him very specific questions. I no longer shot milk across the room when he nursed, and the feeling of my letdown had gone from shooting pains to just a dull sensation.

"Callum, is there still milk in there?"

"Yes."

"Does it taste good?" This question resulted in a sort of puzzled look, like he hadn't really considered it any more.

Later in the pregnancy, my milk dried up completely. I thought this might be the end, but he kept on nursing many times a day: first thing in the morning, whenever he needed the time out from his busy life, and at bedtime. When I asked him if there was milk, he said yes. It's possible that he was able to express some when I wasn't, but I'm pretty sure there was nothing left in there. He seemed sort of anxious when I asked the question, so I told him: *"I don't care if there's milk in there or not. You can keep on nursing."* This seemed to put him at ease, and he admitted that there was no milk.

Sometimes, I was sore, very sore. I had to start saying no to his requests. It was difficult, but now that he was more verbal, we could have really in-depth conversations about this. There were many tears, but eventually, we came to an understanding. He knew that I would never deny him in moments of emotional distress, but still, he missed some of the closeness we always had.

He came up with a charming suggestion one day, *"Mom, can I hold your breast?"* So this is what we worked out, my verbal preschooler and I. Sometimes, when he still needed that time out, but my breasts were sore, he would just hold them. It was sweet and gentle and all his idea.

After a few months of dry nursing, when I was in my eighth month of pregnancy, I noticed him starting to need to swallow more often again, so I asked him again, *"Callum, is there milk in there?"*
"Yes."
"What does it taste like?"

He didn't answer. It was a confusing question, so I clarified, *"Does it taste sweet like ice cream? Or salty like popcorn?"*
"Salty, like popcorn!"
"Is it yummy?"
"No, it's yucky."

At this revelation, I tried not to act too sad or disappointed.
"You don't like it?"
"Yes! I like it! It's good!" he said, and he resumed nursing.

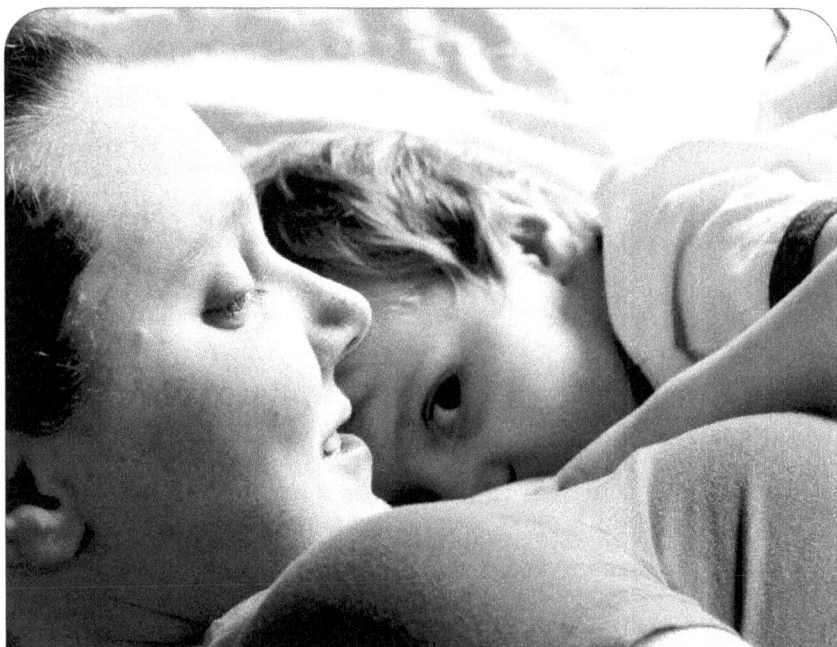

Callum's last nursing session as an only child. It was a special moment that Olivia says she will never forget.

After his sister Lucy was born and my milk came in full swing, we talked a lot about nursing. He told me now that it tasted sweet like ice cream and that, yes, he still liked it. We started to play a game about hypothetical choices:

"Pizza or breast milk?"—*"Breast milk!"*

"Peanut butter sandwich or breast milk?"—*"Breast milk!"*

"Ice cream or breast milk?"—*"Ice cream!"*

"Chocolate or breast milk?"—*"Breast milk!"*

"Slugs or breast milk?"—*"Breast milk!"*

"Popcorn or breast milk?"—*"Popcorn!"*

"Popcorn or ice cream?" That one stumped him.

"Strawberries or breast milk?"—*"Breast milk!"*

To this day, popcorn and ice cream are the only foods that he'd choose over my breast milk. This, of course, makes me feel like a million bucks. Now that my milk was plentiful once again, I grew curious about what his favorite part of breastfeeding was. Surely he must be loving the milk itself. *"No,"* he told me, *"I like the way it feels in my mouth."* This certainly explained why he persevered through those months without milk. Milk was not the most important part of the equation.

Lucy is 2 months old, and Callum grows more articulate and expressive every day. I often have to cut his nursing sessions short to tend to Lucy or to make sure there is enough milk for her. He is very gracious about this.

I think he can tell that I'm a little sad to ask him to let go. So now, when his sessions are over, he'll kiss me and say *"I love you"* or, my favorite, *"I saved some for Lucy!"* Through our conversations and through all those times, he still comes to me crying: *"Want to nurse! Want to nurse!"* I know why he, my giant 3-year-old, needs to nurse. It really hasn't changed. He nurses to eat. He nurses to be healthy. He nurses to feel safe. He nurses to be close to my heart. Only now, he can tell me.

Read more of Olivia's story in Chapters 3 and 5, where she talks about tandem nursing and nursing through mental health concerns.

Magical Mama More
Kirsten Williams, Bethlehem, Pennsylvania

When I was pregnant, one of the few things that I knew was that I would breastfeed. Like any pregnant woman in the United States, I was bombarded with unsolicited advice, horror stories, and rules of parenting, most of which were complete hogwash. When a coworker learned that I planned on breastfeeding to at least 1, she was horrified and said I had to stop at 6 months. I don't think that I discussed parenting issues with her again after that statement.

My own mother-in-law prefaced every single breastfeeding discussion with *"if you can."* I was surrounded by formula-feeding mothers comparing powder dispensers and bottle types. In spite of all this, I just held firmly to my belief that breastfeeding would be a major part of my life as a mother. I knew that if I had confidence in myself and my body, it would work.

I was blessed to have the complete support of my immediate family. My parents wanted the best for their grandchild and their daughter, and never made me feel anything other than comfortable breast-feeding in their presence. My husband was also totally supportive of my desire to breastfeed our child. He did initially have some idea that it should stop after two years. Luckily for the both of us, when that magic age arrived, he saw no reason to take away something so powerful, beneficial, and soothing. Particularly in battling temper tantrums and emotional meltdowns, the soothing power of *"mama more,"* as my daughter calls it, was undeniable, not to mention her health and lack of sick-baby doctor visits.

As my daughter grew from an infant into a toddler and then, seemingly overnight, to a little girl, the moments that she needed to be connected to me physically diminished. I was faced with the combined joy and sadness of watching my wildflower child explore the world and find her own personhood separate from mama. I am so proud to watch her interact with the people and animals that she meets and to see how outgoing and articulate she is, but I miss those long hours of holding her tiny body against mine, feeling like I was still her entire universe, even though she was no longer inside me. When she was breastfeeding, either as an infant, a toddler, or a little girl, that connection was solidified.

I always think of a quote by Elizabeth Stone that is shared often among the *"mommy boards"* that I've been part of since having Veronica: *"Making the decision to have a child—it is momentous. It is to decide forever to have your heart go walking around outside your body."*

In the months surrounding Veronica's third birthday, so many things were happening in our lives. She met her great-grandfather on my mother's side for the first time, I briefly held a full-time job, and her grandmother on her father's side died. This was a stressful and tumultuous time for all of us. There was a lot of travel, she was in daycare for several weeks, and she had to come with me to a memorial about a week and a half after her own birthday.

The day of the memorial, in particular, will stand out forever in my memory as she was surrounded by people she didn't know, in rooms crackling with emotion. I was exhausted after spending most of the previous night awake in my in-laws' apartment waiting for the call from the hospice and then helping my husband and father-in-law get through the day. We were in a sitting room on a little couch, just the two of us, while everyone milled around, ate, shared stories, and readied themselves for the memorial service that my father-in-law had planned. Veronica cuddled into my lap and asked for mama more. As people left the room and filed into the chapel for the service, she and I sat cuddling on the couch as she nursed, wrapped in my arms, just the two of us stealing a moment of serenity. In just minutes, her body relaxed and her breathing deepened, and she fell into the blissful deep sleep of a completely contented child. I carried her into the chapel to join my husband, his family, and their friends to memorialize my daughter's grandmother, and she slept through the entire event.

In addition to practicing full-term breastfeeding, I also bed-share with my daughter, and this has more than likely helped to maintain our breastfeeding relationship. For the last year, I have worked part-time at night, and come home when she should be going to sleep. Every night that I work, my husband starts the bedtime routine with teeth brushing, and face washing, and stories and cuddles, and then I come home and crawl into bed with her for singing and mama more. Some nights, when I come through the door, I hear her jump out of bed, and she runs to me for a hug or a kiss, or grabbing my shirt and lifting it, she will try to get directly to my breasts for a quick nurse before she hops back into bed and waits for me to come for our cuddles. Every morning when she wakes up, she snuggles up next to me and, without opening her eyes, finds my breast to start her day with breastfeeding. I love these moments of just-us time. They center me as much as they provide her with comfort and routine.

I have that bliss of just being with her and shutting out the rest of the world for a few precious moments. Before bed and before we start the day, we connect, the world falls away, and nothing else matters. I cannot express how magical a time that is for me.

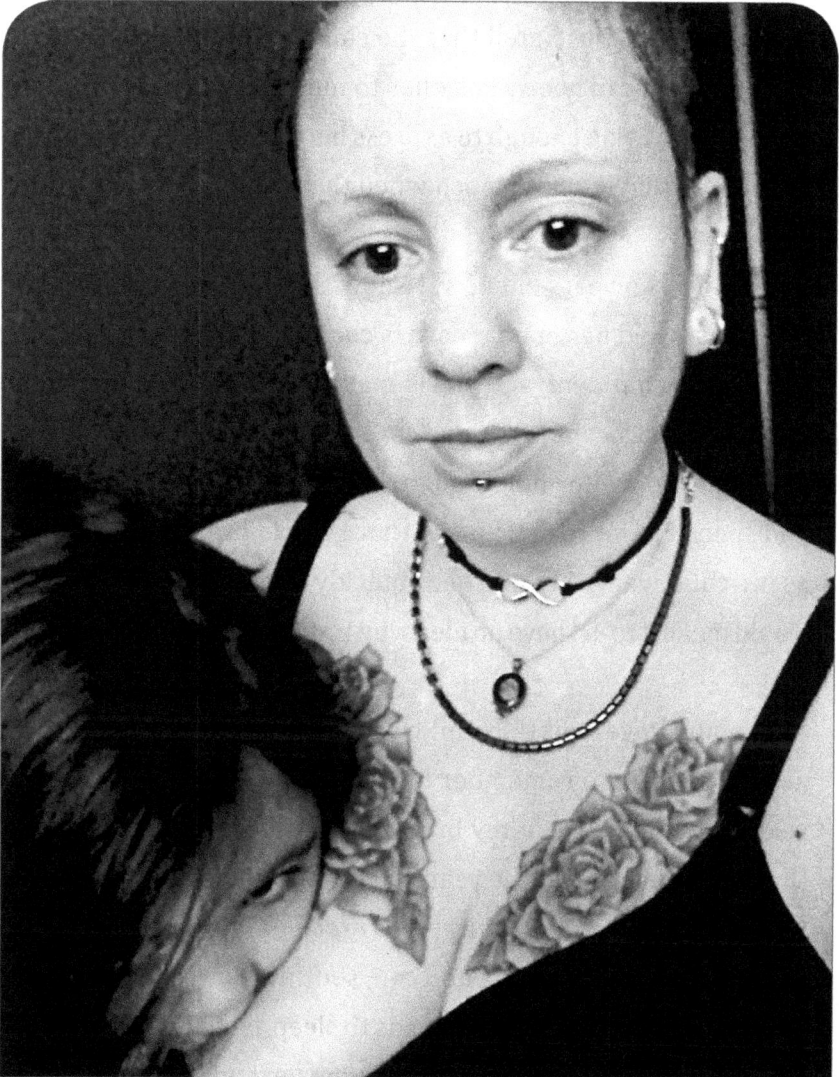

Kirsten and Veronica taking a moment.

This summer, she skinned her knee in our driveway and, howling in pain and surprise, grabbed for my breasts as I cuddled her in front of our house and lifted my shirt so she could soothe herself. In moments, she was calm enough for me to carry her inside to clean and bandage the wounded knee, and then she was off playing again. When she is so frustrated that she can do nothing but curl up in a ball and cry, I can gently coax her to me to sit in my lap and nurse until she can relax enough to express herself, and let go of the anger or sadness that hurts so much when the world is so big.

Veronica is 4 years old now. I know that the time of her needing my breasts and her mama more is coming to an end. She is strong, smart, and confident, and she is making her way and finding new methods to feel connected and soothed. I cradle the moments that she comes to me for nursing like I cradle her body—close, sacred, and special to my heart. I knew that I would breastfeed for as long as my child wanted to and very quickly hoped and prayed that we would make it to 4. I have no idea why I latched onto that age, but I did.

So many have said that children should be weaned before they are old enough to remember breastfeeding. I hope that Veronica remembers her time at my breasts and the warmth, love, and fun that we have had over the years. Here we are, just months after her fourth birthday, still catching those precious moments to connect in the way only mother and child can, soothing ourselves in a primal, ancient, and natural way that leads to sleep, laughter, or just a quick *"love you"* before she scampers off to the next adventure.

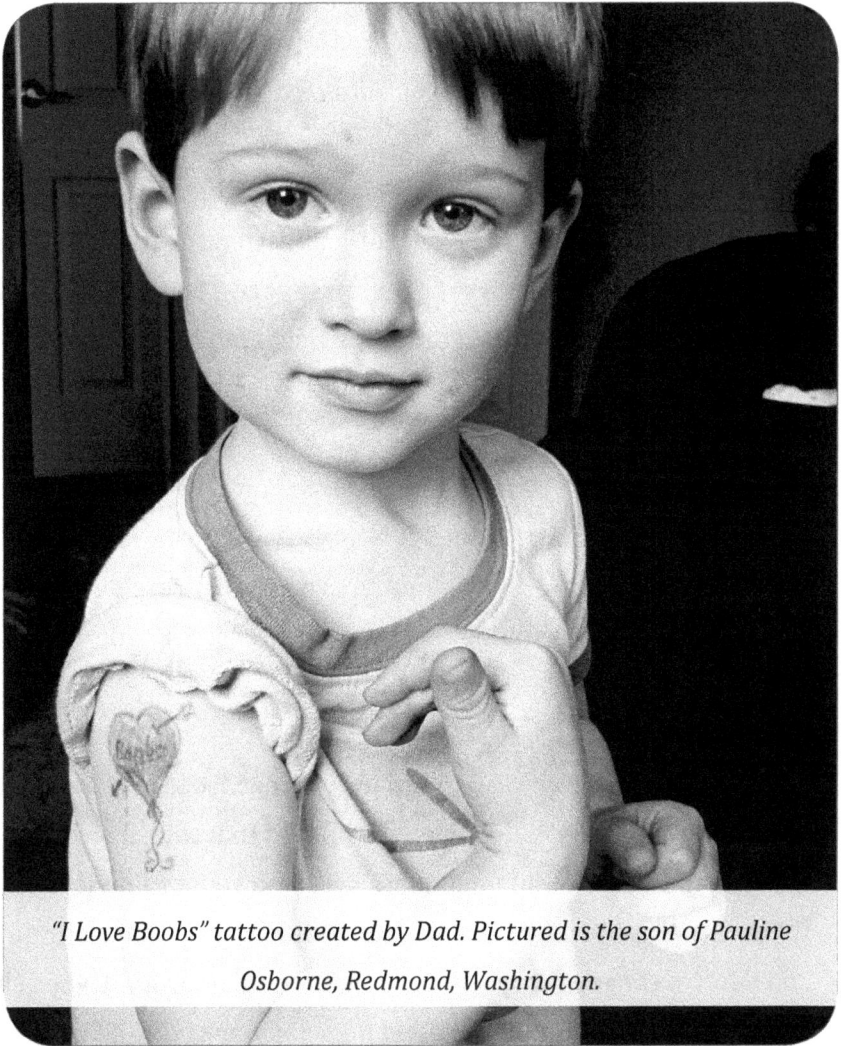

"I Love Boobs" tattoo created by Dad. Pictured is the son of Pauline Osborne, Redmond, Washington.

Just recently, my husband and son Adrian were having a conversation and my son asked how chocolate milk was made. My husband jokingly replied, *"The cows eat chocolate."*

Knowing that I don't like it, Adrian then said, *"Can we get mom to eat chocolate?"*

—Pauline Osborne, Redmond, Washington

Honoring Mommy's Milk
Jackie Bredl-Dietrich, Wisconsin Rapids, Wisconsin

I n two days, my daughter will turn 5½ years old. This is the first time that we've actually paid significant attention to the halfway mark of a year other than that of her first year. There is one reason why this has become important. She has been breastfeeding all this time. With a rough beginning that included difficulty with her latching on followed by sore nipples because my daughter was slightly tongue-tied, for the first month I wondered how new mothers stayed the course with breastfeeding. It was difficult, tiring, and painful. After about four weeks, we turned a corner by addressing the tight frenulum, and breastfeeding shifted into a peaceful, loving, bonding dream between my daughter Josie and me.

I rarely pumped, except when I knew that I needed to be at a meeting or for my own comfort. However, the bottles that she received from her dad and other family members could be counted on less than 10 fingers. Our breastfeeding relationship began to shape our days and how I arranged my schedule so that I could be around when she wanted what would soon be called her *"mommy's milk."* She turned 2, then 3. I never even gave it a thought to stop. It had become a part of our life—the check-in and reenergizing session during the day, the reconnection at the end of the day, the greeting each morning, and the comfort and closeness in the dark night.

As a tiny baby, she very quickly established where she wanted her feet to be. I would hold them in my hand, and she would press gently against it. If they were left unheld, she would find a place to rest them—my belly and, when she grew, my upper thighs—and bounce them up and down rhythmically.

Friends and family checked in at various points to ask something that I never even thought about: *"Are you still breastfeeding Josie?"* and *"When will you stop?"* I always replied with a thoughtful, *"Yes,"* and then said that I was trusting my intuition and going with what felt right for us.

Admittedly, I did envy the moms that took trips without their babies at 6 or 9 months, and I wished that her daddy and other family members could have experienced feeding her with a bottle. I knew that I felt exhausted at times, and breaks were often few and far between. However, the energy exchange with my little girl cuddled tight with her feet tucked in such a way on my upper thighs wasn't something that I would trade. There were times when she was on overload and moving into a negative mood. I would invite her to have some mommy's milk wherever we could find a quiet, private space—just her and me, reconnecting, reassuring, nourishing each other with love and comfort and with confidence. She would look at me with droopy eyes and say, *"Yes, I'd like some mommy's milk."* Then, at some point, she would perk up, shift into a beaming, bright, happy little person again, and be on to her next adventure.

I became pregnant the month following Josie's second birthday. My husband, John, and I were excited and told many people the instant that we found out. Having had a healthy pregnancy and homebirth with Josie, we were optimistic and confident about our second pregnancy. It was perfect timing, or so we thought.

However, 10 weeks into the pregnancy, I had a pregnancy loss. It was a sad, empty time, and I was so grateful that Josie and I never skipped a beat with breastfeeding.

I believe that it's the one thing that eased me through this loss, allowed me to honor it, and trust what was to be. All that I knew is that when I cuddled with my daughter, despite my tears, her tenderness reminded me to be present and enjoy the moment: right then, right there. It offered me a closeness that, admittedly, was difficult for me and my husband as we both journeyed through our grief in different ways. Our dog had also died earlier that year.

Five months after I miscarried, we ended up getting a new puppy and also found out that I was pregnant! This pregnancy went smoothly, and nine months later on a new moon, our baby boy was welcomed into the world.

When I discovered that I was pregnant again, Josie was 2½, and she remained a little being everconnected to her mommy, mommy's milk, and the growing life inside me. We watched videos of babies being born, read birth stories, and talked about what the birth and life with a new baby would be like. She attentively followed my body through its many changes. She eagerly charted my progress and found the baby's heartbeat at our midwife appointments. It was a time to be cherished.

Popular American breastfeeding standards would say that it was way past time for this little girl to stop breastfeeding. She was almost 3, and her mother had endured a miscarriage and was now pregnant.

Her mother's milk must be dried up, so what was the point? Who does that? Isn't it strange?

Being that I was already *"weird"* for having a homebirth and not vaccinating, I didn't see any reason why I should balk at what now would be called extended breastfeeding. So the journey continued through my pregnancy. During the birth, which lasted a span of 22 hours or so, Josie was right there by my side, along with John, my mom, and our midwives. When the time came to go into the birthing tub, Josie eagerly jumped in to swim. She wondered when the baby would be there and asked over and over again. Having a slowly progressing labor was a totally different experience for me than her wild and furious 7-hour birth, and it was a testament to just how patient I'd become.

At one point, we wanted to encourage things along a bit, and I remembered that nipple stimulation aided with this. So, while in the birth tub with our swim suits on, I invited Josie to breastfeed. She was surprised, I think, that I wanted to offer milk to her, and also obliged instantly as if she knew that everyone would benefit. So, in the tub and between contractions, she breastfed as our midwife looked on with a gentle smile. She said, *"It's wonderful that you're breastfeeding Josie and even better right now—just might do the trick."* Afterward, she credited the breastfeeding for moving the birth along and was very proud of us.

Our baby boy latched on instantly, and it was a dream. I thought, *"Wow, this is how it's supposed to work."* There was no soreness and no major engorgement. I knew how to hold him and what his cues were. I was still in the groove, and we started breastfeeding with a running start.

Josie had to learn to share with her new little brother, Trey, and I couldn't think of a better way than for her to share her much-coveted mommy's milk. From what I remember, we made sure that her brother always got what he needed first. It really didn't take long for her to understand, and for many, many months, she savored the fresh supply that her new brother generated. It was like the faucet had been turned on again. She grew like a weed during this time, and neither of them was ever sick except for the occasional cold.

Josie thought for some time that she should breastfeed every time that Trey did, and she would be on one side and Trey on the other, both of them in heaven. As they continued to grow, they would tandem-nurse, hold hands, poke at each other, tickle, bop, kick, and bump; this was most often followed by giggles and milk dribbling off of their lips.

Trey is now just over 2, and Josie will be 5½ in two days. We've had conversations about weaning at the four-year mark and maybe at other trivial times in between. We are always trying to gauge where we both are emotionally and physically with this big commitment that we have made. There are days here and there when she doesn't ask, or even think about, mommy's milk. Then, there are days when she begs and wants to crawl on my lap and does. I say no sometimes, and I say yes sometimes. Most often, she respects my request. It's been nice to be able to talk to her to find out what she likes about mommy's milk. She always just says, *"I like the way it tastes."* I ask her to tell me more and how it tastes; she says, *"It's sweet,"* and that's about all I get.

Postscript

At some point, Josie stopped having mommy's milk altogether. It was such a gradual transition: when I realized it, it had been several days since she had breastfed. I wish that I could tell you exactly how old she was, but I can't. I wrote the previous paragraphs as a way for me to transition and honor the years of breastfeeding moments that I will always cherish with my daughter.

As I write this, Trey is wrapping up his own journey with breastfeeding. He is 5 years old, and most days go by without even a mention of what he fondly refers to as *"milky."* When he does, it is a very short session, almost as if he's just checking things out to see if everything still works. He tells me it does and also states, *"Mommy's milk is yummy, warm, and I like it."* Breastfeeding Trey has been like second nature, and I've done it more comfortably and confidently. When he was little, he went on many family adventures, and I'm thrilled to report that breastfeeding during kayaking can most certainly be accomplished!

I know that for some, it may be a challenge to wrap your thoughts around extended breastfeeding as my family has experienced it. I am very thankful to my husband, John, and my mom, Etta, who because of their support, have offered me the opportunity to be with my children in a consistent way that allowed me to continue breastfeeding. I had a great support team, trusted my body, and followed my heart. We did what felt right for our family.

Today, it is connected hugs, warm cuddles, and honest sharing with my children that are slowly but surely taking the place of mommy's milk or milky. It is not loss that I feel, but instead, I am experiencing a tremendous amount of peace because of the gift of love and closeness that we have shared.

We are at peace. Breastfeeding my children has been a blessing to my life and theirs. I am extremely grateful.

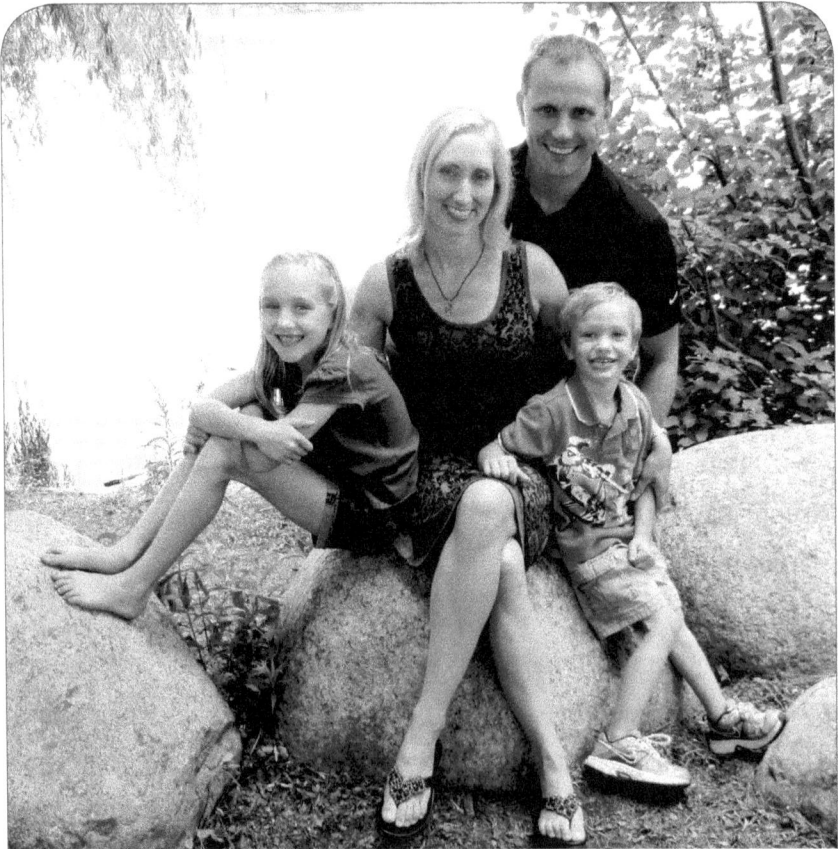

Jackie, John, Josie, and Trey.

Finding Our Place

Shawnee Carini, The Mountains of Northern California

My name is Shawnee. I am 38 years old and the mother of five children (Martin, 11; Hayden, 9; Arabella, 7; Vincent, 3; and Azzurra, 3 months). I started breastfeeding 11 years ago, and I have been breastfeeding continuously for the past 9½ years. All of my children nursed until they were at least 2, and my oldest daughter nursed until she was almost 4.

Breastfeeding has been an unexpected blessing in my life. I always knew that I would breastfeed because it was best for the baby, but I never considered what a gift it would be for me too. I also never considered just how long this journey would last.

I learned early in my journey that for me, child-led nursing schedules and weaning worked best for me and my kids. When my firstborn Martin was 10 months old, I became pregnant. Marty was strictly breastfed at that point, and he weighed 26 pounds. All of my doctors were telling me to wean him because he obviously didn't need it anymore, and that it would take nutrition from me and the new baby.

I didn't listen. I kept on feeding him through the whole pregnancy. My nipples were very tender, and I would have to brace myself before every latch-on. The day Hayden was born, my husband felt that Marty was a *"big boy"* now and should be weaned immediately off the boob. I tried to appease my husband at first, but both Marty and I were miserable, and my heart was breaking. It was causing friction between my husband and me, but I just couldn't let it go.

I felt that if Marty still needed it, and I still wanted to give it to him, then we should be able to do that. Still, over the next week, every family member had an opinion on the subject, and they were making me feel selfish and guilty.

Finally, I called La Leche League. They gave me the number of a local mother and guidance person to talk to. I called her, and we talked for an hour. She was really informative and gave me perspective on the situation. I told her how big Marty was, and how everybody thought he was too big to still need to breastfeed. She told me about a list that gives 100 reasons why children breastfeed, and how nutrition was only one of them. She told me about breastfeeding and its culture from all over the world.

After that conversation, I realized that child-led breastfeeding and weaning were what made sense for me. The last thing I was going to do was conform to some rule that society chose for me. Why exactly was it not acceptable for me to nurse my toddler and my newborn together? Why does everyone in society seem supportive about breastfeeding and then glare at you when you are in public breastfeeding your 1-year-old?

At last, I did not care what other people thought. From that day on, I tandem-nursed my newborn and almost-toddler for a year. It became the beginning of 10 years of breastfeeding adventure.

When Arabella was born, Hayden had just turned 2. About a week after she was born, he just didn't want the boob anymore. From the moment Arabella started breastfeeding, she was in baby heaven.

Now, all of my children loved breastfeeding, but there was something even more special about her connection. Every time she saw a boob, or I laid her down in position, she would get happy. Then, when she started feeding, it was like her whole energy shifted.

She went from being a happy baby to a blissful baby. She exuded joy out of every pore of her being. She was happy, peaceful, contented, and getting filled with milk. It was not just her belly being filled, but her soul too. As her mother, I was happy for her and so glad to be sharing this experience with her. She was just a little baby at that point, but over the course of our almost four years of breastfeeding experience together, her joy never really ceased. She was always happy concerning the subject and never whined like some of my kids when they wanted it. She was elated all the time. It brought her joy well into her fourth year. As she got older, her feedings were mainly at night. She was so active during the day, as most 3-year-olds are, that she only slowed down enough for nursing in the evening.

A memorable moment for me was on her third birthday. We had invited our neighbors over for cake and tea, and our guests were just arriving. Arabella was having a great time. Dressed in cowgirl boots and her birthday tutu, she was ready to roll, and roll she did, right off our loft ladder with a hard thud to the ground. She had a rather bad bump on her head. We did the normal first-aid care, but she was very distraught. An ice pack, arnica remedy, and rescue remedy were helping her body, but she needed something more. So, we nursed there on the couch. I nursed her for 2 hours, singing to her, reading to her, and trying to keep her awake for fear that she might have a concussion.

I remember thinking how special and convenient it was to have a built-in comforting tool. She lay there, and I lay there, as we were both comforted by breastfeeding. I realized how comforting it was for me to be able to provide her some healing in that scary moment. As a mother, it was the one go-to method I had that would always work. It was like magic, a magic potion flowing from my breasts that would always provide whatever was needed. Whether it was for food, security, or comfort, it was always there.

When Arabella was just shy of her fourth birthday, she stopped nursing, but even though she had stopped breastfeeding, she was still so happy anytime she saw my breasts. She would get a look of happiness on her face. Four months after she weaned, I became pregnant with my fourth child.

When I was about seven months pregnant (a year after Bella had weaned herself), we were in the shower together. She was looking at me and said, *"Oh, Mama, those boobs look so big and beautiful. I wanna suck that sweet, sweet milk out of them."*

For me, these were words that I will never forget; they were so sweet and off the cuff. A year after she had stopped breastfeeding, she still felt fondly about it. After I had the baby, she asked me for a taste, and I gave it to her. Although she liked the taste, she had outgrown the need to breastfeed.

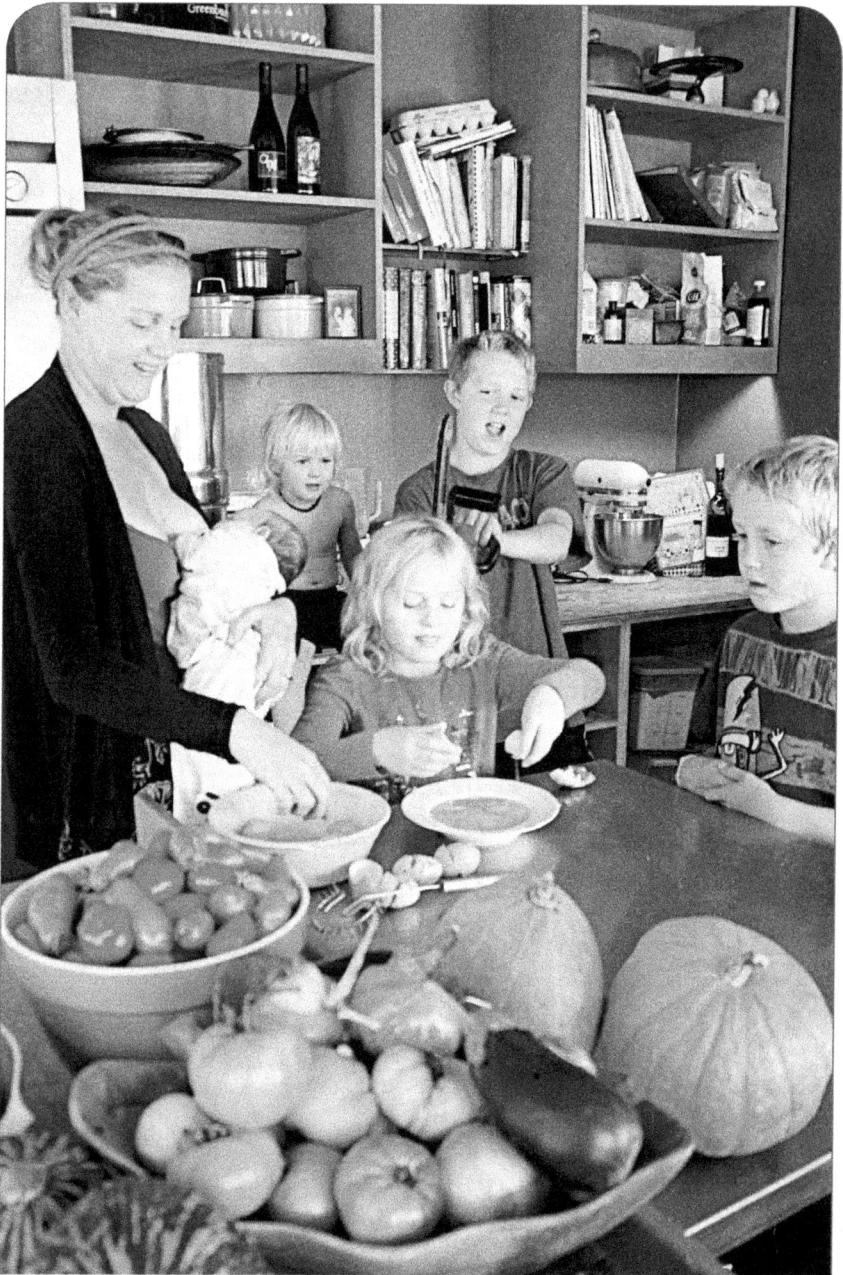

*Shawnee multitasking with her
five children as she nurses the youngest.*

In the end, when I followed my heart and my intuition and stood up for what I believed in, everyone around me followed suit. Eleven years, nine and a half years of breastfeeding, and five kids later, I feel supported by my husband and all those around me. My husband doesn't blink an eye anymore at a public feeding, and if the public doesn't like it, they can look away. Maybe it's because I don't take no for an answer. I do what I need to do when and where I need to do it. I feel strong in my ability to listen to my children, even from infancy, about their needs concerning breastfeeding. They are very smart, those little people. They are very good about giving me signs of when, how much, and how long they will be on this journey with me. They call the shots (within reason). I just try to have an open heart and listen to them. After all, this is a gift that we are giving to each other. A precious and most important gift of life, patience, and love.

Where We Are

Some say I should have walls around me and a
door closed. I think we should just be where we are.
These are the places I've breastfed my babies...

On the side of the road,

the county fair,

at a school recital,

my cozy bed in the wee hours of the morning and night,

parent–teacher conferences,

California, Michigan, Nevada,

Kopp's Custard in Milwaukee, Wisconsin,

Disneyland,

the airport lobby,

standing in a security line, an airplane,

at the dinner table,

and under the shade of an oak tree.

We've nursed on the couch snuggly warm,

around the bonfire,

10th row at a Phish show,

in the garden,

at the grocery store,

in the shower,

Thanksgiving dinner,

in my kitchen,

in the woods hauling wood,

at work,

on the toilet,

my cousin's funeral, and

Uncle Christian's wedding.

The babies have grown inch by inch as we

breastfeed wherever

we go;

Spain,

Italy,

a fallen down coliseum pillar in Rome,

the Parthenon in Athens, Greece,

black volcanic beach on Santorini Island,

Aunt Bridgett's high school graduation,

Thai restaurant in Kalamazoo with the good

pad thai,

and by the side of the Trinity River.

Whether we are out and about or at our house,

we breastfeed wherever we are.

Getting Out of the Way and Letting It Work
Lara Audelo, Colorado, Springs, Colorado[4]

As I sit down and write this, I have been breastfeeding for exactly six-and-a-half years. With my first son Owen, I set a goal for breastfeeding while I was pregnant, but I had no idea what to expect when it came to the realities of breastfeeding. Thankfully, we enjoyed a beautiful nursing relationship that came to a close when he was 27 months old. I really wanted to breastfeed him until his second birthday, and when he weaned, I was six months pregnant with his little brother. I was so happy that we had achieved my goal and was thankful for the confidence that breastfeeding gave me in all areas of motherhood.

There's a certain amount of trust that a breastfeeding mother has to have in her body, as you kind of have to get out of the way for it to work properly. If you try to measure, schedule, or regulate too much, it just doesn't work as it's supposed to. That trust taught me how to really tune into my body, and that led to me being able to do the same for my intuition. Just as I followed my instincts when it came to breastfeeding, it felt right to do the same in other aspects of parenting. For me, this meant a great deal of physical closeness with Owen, such as we experience with bed sharing and baby wearing, without the unfounded fear that keeping him close would spoil him, as many tried to suggest.

When my younger son Foster was born, he started nursing immediately. Four years and three months later, we are still bonding

---

4   Lara Audelo is the author of *The Virtual Breastfeeding Culture: Seeking Mother to Mother Support in the Digital Age* (Praeclarus Press, 2013).

through breastfeeding. I had the same initial goal for him as I did with Owen: I wanted us to reach the two-year milestone. When Foster was an infant, I had doubts that we would make it that long because he was so busy and curious and constantly on the go. I wondered if he would separate from me sooner than his brother and just lose interest in the breast. When his second birthday arrived, I celebrated once again because we had met the goal! I exhaled a little and just adopted the attitude that I would let him decide when he was ready to wean without pressuring him.

At 2, he still breastfed often: every morning, a couple times during the day, including to sleep for his nap, at bedtime every night, and then during the night. Bed sharing made it very easy for him to continue breastfeeding during the night, and it was never bothersome to me because he would just want to nurse briefly, and then he'd be back to sleep in no time. Of course, the morning nursing session in bed meant that I could stay asleep, or pretend to be asleep, for a little longer, so maybe that was more for me than for him! At 4 years old, he nurses in the morning when we wake, at night before bedtime, and occasionally during the day if we have a chance or if he is feeling a little puny or under the weather.

Ages 2 and 3 can be challenging for kids and parents. Having experienced this stage with my older son, I knew what was coming as Foster grew older.

The natural tendency for a child is to become physically independent. It starts when he crawls and walks, and as he grows, he ventures farther and farther away. However, that exploration, while exciting and stimulating for him, can be tough and can leave him with a strong need to still be physically connected to his mother for security. When this discovery process was happening and Foster was pushing the boundaries of his comfort zones, I found breastfeeding to be the best tool in my parenting toolkit.

When he was 3, I oftentimes used breastfeeding as a way to calm and comfort him; it seemed to nourish his spirit more than his body. The fact that he was receiving breast milk that was changing just as he was through the years and was providing him with nutritional and immunological benefits was kind of an ancillary bonus. Scientific studies have shown that breastfeeding is the perfect food for a child's growing brain, which as we know develops rapidly from birth to age 5. Mother Nature has matched children's physiological need for breast milk with the ability of the process to nurture them emotionally as they play, explore the world, and acquire independence. Having the perspective of six-and-a-half years as a breastfeeding mother, I can truly appreciate this amazing system. Ask any mom who breastfeeds a 3-year-old what the best way to calm her tired, frustrated child is, and she will tell you a warm lap, a pair of loving arms, and some breast milk. It doesn't get any easier for the mother or her child.

On another note, I must say that the little things that a nursing preschooler says to his or her mother can put a smile on anyone's face. On various occasions, Foster has convinced me to sit down and take a little nursing break with reminders such as, *"Mommy, your milk has special vitamins for me."* This proves that little children really do listen because I am pretty sure I know where he heard that statement. He doesn't stop there though, as many times while nursing, he uses his vivid imagination and says, *"This side tastes like coffee, and that side tastes like chocolate milk!"* Perhaps my favorite times are when he asks to nurse and I try to delay him because I am in the middle of something; he will say, *"Just five sips, Mommy!"*

It is normal to nurse a 4-year-old, but it is just uncommon in our society. So telling people that he still breastfeeds at age 4 is always a little interesting because the looks on people's faces are priceless. It doesn't come up in conversation often, but if it does, I don't hide the fact, and I go so far as to share why I still breastfeed and the benefits of full-term breastfeeding. With my firstborn, I was much less forthcoming about some aspects of my parenting style. Even though they felt right for me, they were not very mainstream. Depending on whose company I was in, I kept quiet about breastfeeding and bed sharing. Now, I have no secrets because I think that it is important that we talk about these aspects of our lives so that others who do the same know that they are not alone in their choices. If I can speak up and help someone feel better and more confident in her choices, I take that opportunity.

I never expected Foster to breastfeed this long, but I am so thankful that he has. What has full-term breastfeeding taught me? I know because of our experience that breastfeeding a 4-year-old is no stranger than breastfeeding a 4-month-old. Different? Yes. There's more in the way of arms and legs to contend with, and a 4-year-old can clearly communicate things, such as which side he wants to nurse on, for how long, and so on, but when my son looks up into my eyes as he rests on my lap and latches on, I'm quickly reminded that those are the same hazel eyes that looked at me when he was 10 minutes old and breastfed for the first time. It is still one of the best ways to calm him and get him to slow down. I have no idea when he will wean, and I know that it will be bittersweet when he just wants snuggles but no more milk. I love that he is now old enough to remember breastfeeding, and I hope that he will cherish these memories for the rest of his life, as I know I will.

Our children come bearing many gifts, which they reveal to us over the course of time, and I know for sure that breastfeeding past the age of 4 is one of Foster's gifts to me.

Nursing as Seen through My Daughter's Eyes
Jessica Fisher, Lakeland, Florida

I keep a small leather-bound journal so that I can record all the sweet, small moments that I might otherwise forget. The sweetest moments I've had with my daughter Claire have been while nursing. While I can think of countless reasons that I enjoy our nursing relationship, seeing it through her eyes has been the biggest reward of all.

When we began, I was committed to breastfeeding until at least age 2 for the health and bonding benefits that I read and heard so much about, but it was Claire herself who convinced me to remain committed to nursing past age 3 and beyond. Claire is now 4 and is as enthusiastic as ever about nursing.

At least a thousand times, I've brought her to my breast while she was hurt or afraid and helped her find comfort in my arms. It feels so powerful to be able to provide such instant and complete security for her and to feel her relax into me. At least a hundred times, I've looked down anxiously at the top of her head, worried about a bumped head or bruised pride, only to hear her sigh and look up at me through tear-stained lashes. It's almost as if I can read her mind, and she is saying, *"Thank you, Mama. I'm better now."*

Nursing always provides complete healing for both of us, no matter what caused the upset. After a few minutes of sitting calmly and nursing, everything seems right with the world again and, more importantly, right between the two of us. As Claire grows and parenting her becomes increasingly complex, I am endlessly grateful for that bond. Thirty seconds of nursing accomplishes more than a thousand words. I am usually at a total loss for words after an intense power struggle or tantrum. Instead, I sit or stand nearby and hold my arms open for her. Without fail, she runs into my arms and finds comfort in nursing after the worst of the tantrum is over.

When Claire was barely 2, we were reading a book about a boy who accidentally hit a baseball through a neighbor's window. The picture showed the angry neighbor about to confront the boy. Claire looked at the picture and said matter of factly, *"Man mad. Man need milka."* I was completely in awe. While it was clear to me that nursing was a critically important part of Claire's process of dealing with difficult emotions, it never occurred to me that she was as equally aware of it.

If she hears a younger baby fussing or crying in public, she frequently will turn her full attention to watch what is happening. Seeing her look of concern, I often ask, *"What do you think is the matter?"* She usually responds, *"That boy wants his mommy milk."*

Recently, I brought out nail polish and pedicure supplies to prepare for a wedding that we were attending. The combination of a 3-year-old and nail polish resulted in a big, fun mess. Claire sprayed me all over with a bottle of fragrant refreshing foot spray. Later, however, when she went to nurse, she got incredibly frustrated, saying, *"Mama! I don't like your smell!"* She tried to latch on repeatedly but then refused. She cried, *"I want you to smell like how your milkas usually smell!"* I have grown to understand that her joy in nursing includes everything about it, not just the milk itself but my scent, the sound of my beating heart, and the feeling of being held in my arms.

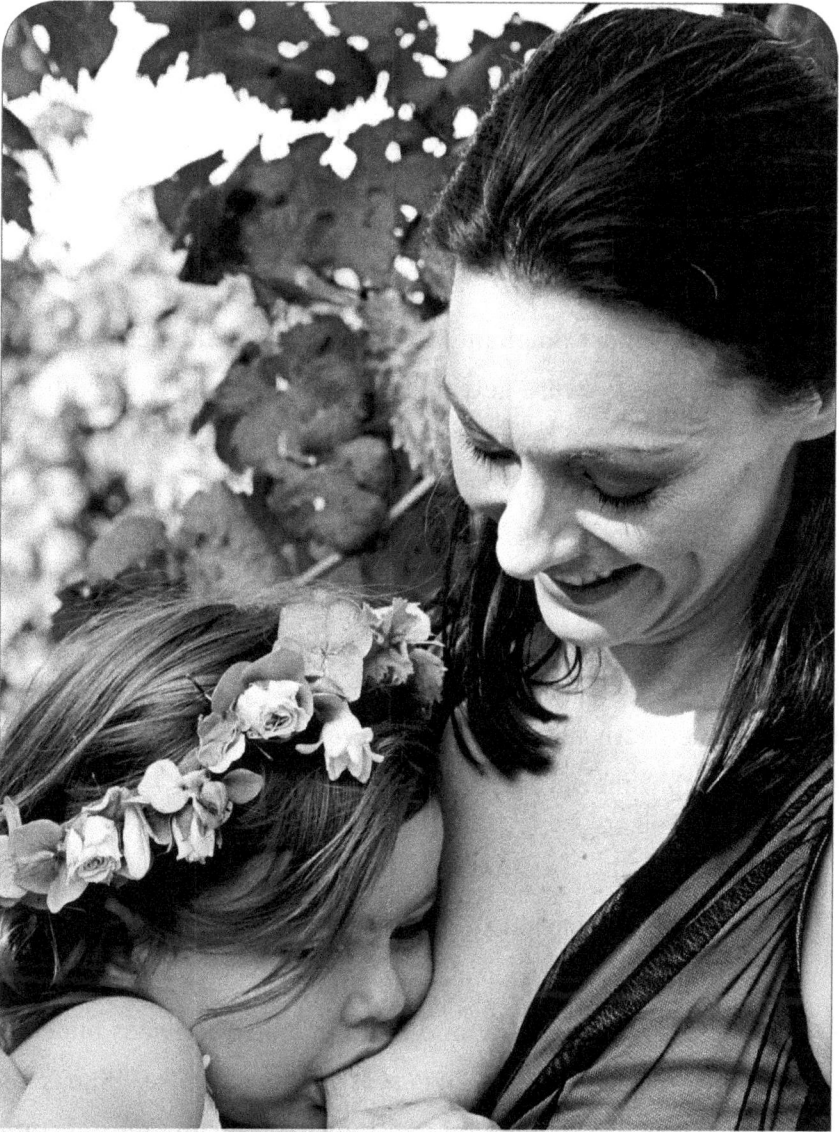

Jessica nursing Claire when she was nearly 4 at a friend's wedding in California. Between jet lag, allergies, and the stress of being a flower girl, Claire needed some comfort from Mommy. Jessica found a place to sit so that their picture could be taken, but under the circumstances, Claire needed to nurse.

She reminded me of this again tonight when she sat in the chair where I had been sitting. She said, *"I want to sit in your chair, Mommy. I like your smell."* Then, coming across the kitchen, she leaned against me as I worked at the counter and said, *"Can I always be close to you, Mama?"*

One of our most poignant moments happened when Claire was about 2½. As we were getting ready for bed, she was exuberant about her *"milkas."* She often does a happy dance when she sees me getting into my nightgown; dancing and running across the bed to me, she flings her arms around me to nurse.

One night, as I started to nurse her, she began singing, *"I love my milkas, I love my milkas!"*

It seemed natural to ask, *"Why do you love your milkas?"*

She simply answered, *"Because I want my mommy,"* and reached for me.

Hilariously, she has told me that my milk tastes like strawberries, cherries, blueberries, and even ice cream. Usually, she reports that it tastes like her favorite food du jour. When she sees me eating something, she often asks, *"Will that go into my milka?"* She is fascinated by the idea that what I eat finds its way into her milk, and I take advantage of the chance to tell her that she is eating kale, sushi, or spicy salsa—anything to encourage a more adventurous palate.

One of the things I like best about nursing Claire beyond 3 years old is that she is very much consciously aware of nursing as a fundamental aspect of mothering. When she plays with her baby dolls, nursing is one of her favorite ways to mother them. I often hear her cooing and talking gently to her dolls, *"It's okay, baby. It's okay. You're a little fussy. I just need to give you a little mommy milk."*

She recently announced, *"When I am bigger, I'm going to be a mommy, and I'm going to have two babies."*

I asked, *"Why will you have two babies?"*

Slightly exasperated by my silly question, she replied, *"Because I have two milkas!"*

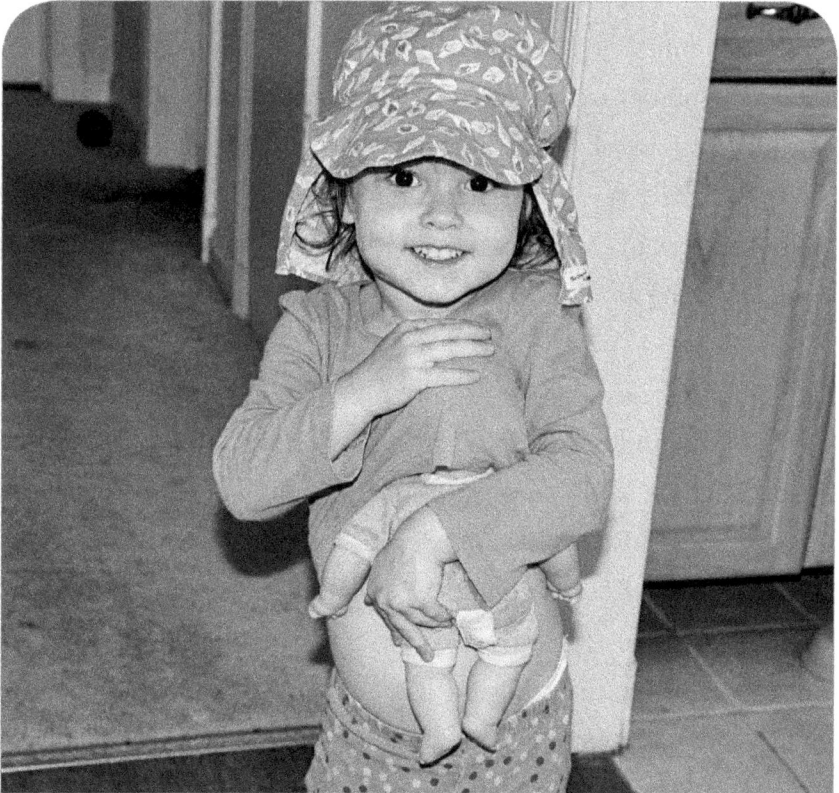

When Claire plays with her baby dolls, she often mothers them by giving them her milkas.

I love the idea that my 4-year-old daughter is not only planning to nurse but that she is planning to tandem-nurse her own children. I also love the idea that she primarily and strongly associates breasts with nursing. In spite of whatever images the media and popular culture will show her about breasts later in life, at least she will have this experience with nursing to balance against those images.

One of my favorite stories occurred when Claire was about 3 years 2 months old. It was Christmas time, and because of my husband's military service, we had shopping privileges at the commissary on the local military base. Not many other people were shopping that evening, and as we walked past Santa and his sleigh, he beckoned to us to come over. Claire had only recently learned about Santa and was intrigued. We approached cautiously, and after I explained what would happen, Claire agreed to sit on his knee and have a photo made as long as I stayed with her holding her hand.

As she sat with Santa, he asked her the usual questions about what she wanted for Christmas and whether she had been a good girl. Then he said, *"Now, on Christmas, I'm going to come to your house and climb down the chimney and bring you toys and leave them under the Christmas tree, but will you please leave me some milk and cookies?"* Claire's eyes grew even wider than they already were, and she looked at me and then back at Santa and then back at me again with a look of complete bewilderment.

The look on her face didn't surprise me, as I knew that the entire experience must seem completely bizarre from her 3-year-old perspective.

Even later that night, I still didn't grasp what was going through her mind. As we were snuggling up to read bedtime stories, she peppered me with questions about Santa. Most of all, she was concerned about his request that she leave him milk and cookies. *"But Mama, why does he want that?"* she asked. I naively replied, *"Well, I guess he just likes milk and cookies."* *"But why does he like that, Mama?"* she asked, incredulously. Because we generally avoided dairy and sweets, I assumed she was concerned that Santa should be making better dietary choices. She said, *"I think we should leave him something else."* After a bit of discussion, we decided that almond milk and raisins would be a better snack for Santa.

It wasn't until a few days later that I fully understood what she had been thinking. We were comfortably rocking and nursing in the nursing rocker when Claire suddenly popped off my breast and looked up with me with pleading eyes and said with great concern, *"But Mama, I don't want to share my milkas with Santa!"*

As what she must have been thinking dawned on me, I worked hard to stifle my giggles. We discussed it, and I learned she had, in fact, thought that Santa was planning on sneaking into her house and wanted to drink her milkas. It finally registered with me why she had such a bewildered look on her face as she kept looking at me and then at Santa and back at me again. Even now that she is a year older, she and I still laugh together about the time when she thought Santa wanted her milkas.

Another funny thing happened when Claire was 3, and she and I were taking a plane trip to Florida. Although I rarely hesitate to nurse in public, I do feel a bit more modest in the close quarters of an airplane. We had the window and middle seats, and I had long since mastered the combination of a nursing tank and a cardigan for modesty. As the engines roared and the plane raced down the runway for takeoff, Claire instinctively reached for me and began nursing. However, as she often does when she is agitated or anxious, she also reached for my other nipple and pulled it out of my shirt so that she could play with it between her fingers as she nursed. This habit is something veteran nursing moms warned me that I should nip in the bud when it began, but I didn't, and so I have just tolerated it all along, even though it can be very, very annoying.

I quickly adjusted the cardigan to cover my other breast and tried to whisper discretely, *"Sweetheart, I don't want everyone to see my private milkas."* Claire responded by shrieking at the top of her lungs, *"But I can't see MY MILKAS!"* *"So much for discretion,"* I thought as every passenger on the plane turned to look at us. There are definitely two of us in this nursing relationship.

The other day, when we were discussing different types of jobs and occupations, she said, *"Mommy takes care of me and gives me milkas."* For her, it is as beautifully simple as that. Having a preschooler who can communicate clearly about nursing is incredible, and I am so grateful to be able to hear directly from my child about what nursing means to her. Nursing to 3 and beyond has allowed me tremendous insight into how passionate and fiercely protective she is of her milkas. As she grows more and more articulate about her love of nursing, I feel tremendously grateful that I have been able to give her this gift.

Memories of Nursing My Children
Debbie Wollensack, Ballarat, Australia

I am at a baby-wearing conference, giving a presentation on do-it-yourself baby carriers. My almost 2-year-old is not happy to sit with Daddy and darts to me and clings to my leg. I quickly offer a cheese stick, but it's no good. I have a ring sling in my hand, so I think, *"Why not?"* I pick him up and pop him in my sling, which calms his restlessness only for a second, so I offer him my breast. He settles immediately and goes to sleep.

When my first child was born over 14 years ago, I could never have imagined breastfeeding a toddler, let alone in front of 20 people! How times change! My son is my fifth breastfed toddler. Looking back, I can't quite believe that I have breastfed without a break for 14 years! It has been an amazing journey. I wasn't sure that I was going to breastfed at all when my first child was born. No one I knew did, and I lived in an area with very low breastfeeding rates. I was lucky to have an amazing general practitioner, who lent me booklets from the Australian Breastfeeding Association. I took them out of politeness at first, but once I actually did read them, I discovered helpful advice and positive messages.

At my first visit with this doctor after my baby was born, I complained that my arms and back got tired from sitting in one spot for so long. She left the room and came back with her old breast-feeding pillow! I felt so fortunate to have met such a great doctor. My son grew into a toddler, and he was eating solid food well but was still devoted to *"milkie."* We were both enjoying it, and I didn't see the need to stop. I felt that since the World Health Organization recommends breastfeeding for at least two years, I had science behind me. My husband was supportive, although every now and then he (and other relatives) would say, *"Isn't he getting too old?"*

I read widely about breastfeeding in other cultures (the world-wide age of weaning is 4!) and was very interested in one study in *Breastfeeding: Biocultural Perspectives* by Katherine A. Dettwyler that compared humans to other animals (see Editor's Note on page #269.) According to Dettwyler, if we look at baby's development and biology and take away the influence of culture, humans would breastfeed for up to seven years.

I was aware that I was doing something unusual in my culture though, so I often reread the books that I had collected. *Mothering Your Nursing Toddler* by Norma Jane Bumgarner was a favorite. Once I had an Internet connection, I frequented forums about breast-feeding and gentle mothering. I used to think about (and talk about and read about) breastfeeding often, but after such a long time, it has faded into the background of my day and only comes to the fore when I hear news stories of discrimination, like a recent one about a breastfeeding mum being asked to cover up at a pool.

I have not experienced much overt discrimination over breast-feeding apart from funny looks or whispers behind hands, and perhaps some of that is more perceived than real. I remember that I was breastfeeding an almost 2-year-old on a bench in the middle of a shopping center—she was desperate and wouldn't be put off—when a woman came up to me. I prepared myself for an attack, but all she said was, *"You're a good mum."* Another time, I was at a presentation dinner, and my toddler was getting restless and was about to cry. *"Feed him!"* insisted a work colleague of my brother. Her favorite footballer was about to make a speech, and she didn't want to miss it!

Once my toddlers were older, they were often too busy to feed much if we were on an outing or out visiting. They still fed a lot at home, but this tapered off gradually until it was just in the morning when they first woke, to fall asleep for naps, after naps, and then at bedtime. When they dropped their naps, it was just at bedtime.

I have fed a child older than 3 only a handful of times in public, more often in front of family or friends, but they know me well and are used to my *"odd"* ways, so they don't bother to say anything anymore and have given up offering a quiet spot in another room. I have always been impressed by my dad, though. If I am feeding a baby or toddler of whatever age, he'll come, sit down, and talk to me. He's not bothered at all.

I was glad to feed my older toddlers in public if needed, but I sometimes found the reactions of others off-putting. I was at a playgroup with my son (in which the dynamics didn't suit me, admittedly, but it was nearby, and my son liked it) when he climbed to the top of a tall slide, suddenly realized how high it was, and was terrified. One of the mums rescued him for me, which he didn't like either. He was so upset that I fed him to comfort and calm him. Never mind that he was 3½. Some of the mums wouldn't speak to me after that, but I just saw it as an excuse to find a better playgroup, and I did. I discreetly fed another son at school pickup time when he was 3 on an out-of-the-way bench, but one of the mums who had been on canteen duty came to give me some change that my son had forgotten and was totally shocked. Every time I saw her after that, she was so nervous that I felt sorry for her. Overall though, on the few times I have fed my older children in public, no one has said anything at all and likely didn't even notice.

I have breastfed through pregnancy and tandem-fed four times. I must admit that I didn't enjoy that as I tended to feel touched out, but I felt that it was such an important transition for them and a source of security. My toddlers were never jealous of their new siblings (although sometimes they were upset with me!).

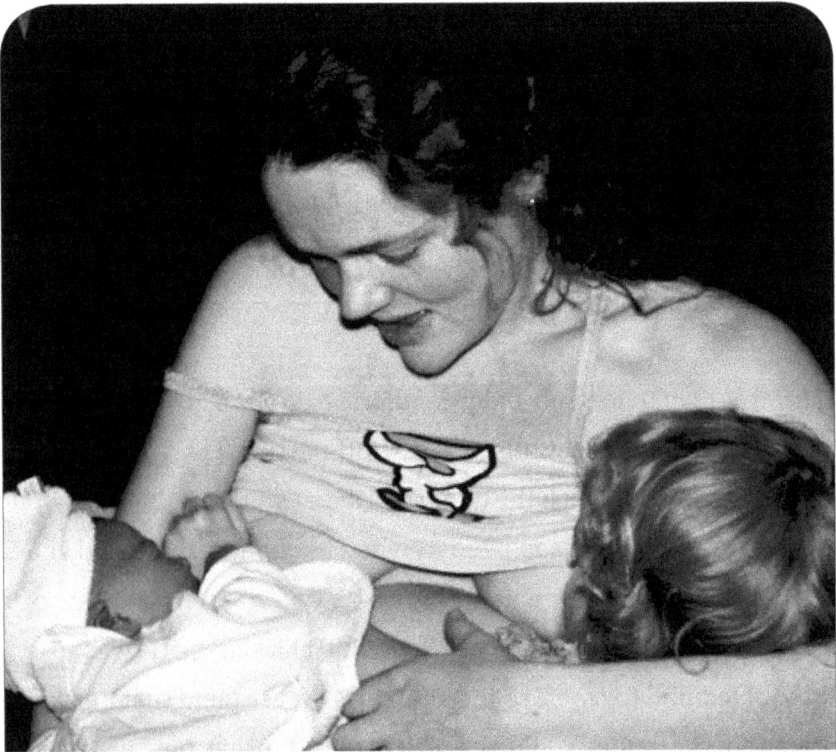

Debbie tandem-nursing her newborn and 3-year-old daughters.

I have fed three children for more than four years (the oldest for four-and-a-half years) and one child for almost three years. She fed about three times once her brother was born but then decided milk was for babies.

I love the closeness of breastfeeding skin to skin: the feel of their warmth and the rise of their breath, how they play with my face and clothes (although I could live without the *"dental exams"*), and the cute things they say.

I once asked my daughter what my milk tasted like.

"Jellybeans!" she declared. Other times, I have been told it's like ice cream or chocolate.

I hope that my children remember being fed. My almost 90-year-old grandma remembers being fed by her mum. As soon as her mother arrived home, she would lead her to her favorite chair, and they would have a feed and cuddle. Her memory is clear and full of affection.

I don't know where my breastfeeding journey with my current nursling will lead, but I'm happy to let him take the lead.

Chapter 3

Making It Work in Everyday Life

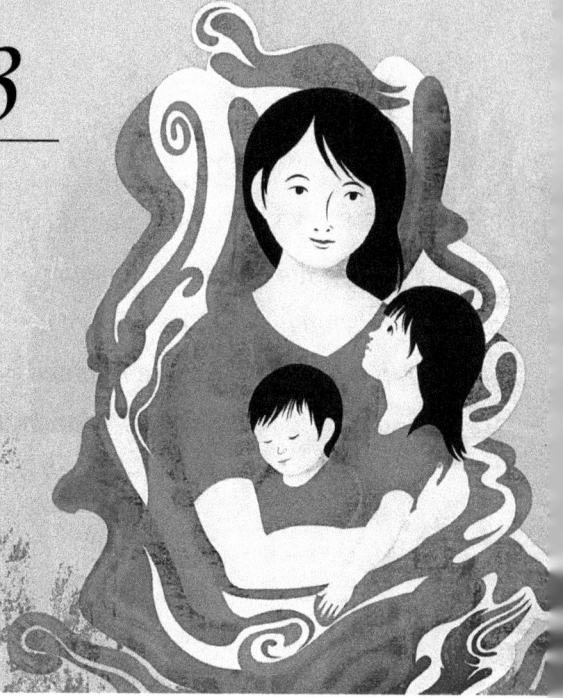

We all have our ways of doing things, and mothering through breastfeeding is no different. Some mothers feel a *"free-for-all"* approach to breastfeeding is best, where the breast is always available—wherever, whenever. Others find that the only way that they can continue to meet their child's needs is to cut back and set limits. In this chapter, you'll find stories of tandem nursing, infertility, and just basic day-to-day life with nurslings that can let Mama know in no uncertain terms whether they still need milk.

"When Sam was 3, he asked to nurse every time he got hurt. When his 6-year-old cousin was visiting, she hurt herself while playing in the barn. I heard her crying and asked Sam what had happened. 'Eleanore bumped her head,' he reported and then added to reassure me, 'Grandma will nurse her.'"

—*Sarah Diener Beachy, Fulks Run, Virginia*

A Solution for Everything
Roberta Samec, Toronto, Ontario, Canada

I remember the first La Leche League (LLL) meeting that I attended when I was pregnant with my first daughter, Isabella. I came with a mission in mind: to learn all that I could about breastfeeding so that I could manage working and nursing when the time came. I own my own business and am, therefore, not entitled to maternity leave benefits. My husband, who can get benefits, was to take the lion's share of the leave and help me with work. I had a goal: to make it to at least a year, ideally to around 15 months or so to get Bella through the worst of cold and flu season. I distinctly remember seeing one of the women at the meeting nurse a small baby and a huge child, who was at least 2 years old. My eyes bugged out, and all I could think about was a sketch from the show *Little Britain,* where a full-grown man is nursing from his mother.

Now, four years later, I'm an LLL Leader, and eyes are bugging out at me while I nurse both my 10-month-old and my nearly 4-year-old. I'm still not sure how I got here.

Nursing was a struggle at the beginning with Bella. It was an uncomplicated pregnancy and quick natural birth with a midwife at St. Michael's Hospital in Toronto at 38 weeks. Then, they weighed Bella: she was only 4 pounds 14 ounces. This triggered a glucose test, and it was determined that she had low blood glucose. There was a transfer of care from our midwife to a neonatal doctor, who determined that Bella should spend some time in the neonatal intensive care unit (NICU) with a glucose drip IV.

The first time she latched well was the evening after she was brought to the NICU, and it was with the help of a lactation consultant. Sadly, this victory was short-lived, as the activity caused the IV in the back of her hand to come out, and blood spurted all over both of us. It was slightly traumatic.

We got through this ordeal with the help of our excellent midwife and the (mostly) helpful staff at the hospital, and Bella was home three days later. One trick that our midwife taught us at the hospital (when Bella was having difficulty with latching) was the use of a makeshift at-breast supplementer, which we continued to use with pumped milk for a while after she got home to help get her weight up.

Working and nursing was tough at times. I work from a home office as a commissioned sales representative for book publishers. For the most part, I control the where and when of my meetings, so my husband Adam and Bella could join me or at least be nearby while I was at meetings.

I have many fond memories of meetings with booksellers with both Adam and the baby there. There was one book fair dinner where the booksellers happily passed Bella around the room. When Adam and Bella couldn't be there, I pumped throughout meetings. This was, without a doubt, the most unpleasant part of nursing, but it was a reminder to myself and those that I was working with that my first priority was the baby at home, who was entirely reliant on me for food. This helped ease my sadness and guilt when we were apart. Nursing was my solution to everything. Hunger, exhaustion, sickness, fear—my solution was always to *"stick a boob in it"* whatever *"it"* was.

When my husband went back to work, Bella was 13 months old. She went to a shared nanny used by one of Adam's coworkers. I didn't pump during the day then (I had had enough of pumping at that point), but nursing was the first thing she did in the morning, when she came home from childcare (which was a great opportunity to put my feet up after a long work day!), and before she went to bed. She was slow to come to solids, but I didn't worry because nursing ensured that she had everything she needed, particularly on days when she was a picky eater or not feeling well. Sick days meant that she would nurse all day, and I knew I was doing the best thing to make her well. I have never fretted about malnutrition or dehydration, and that's all thanks to breastfeeding.

Fifteen months came and went, and this relationship continued, even when she started taking to solids with gusto. She started to talk, and suddenly, we had a name for nursing: *"side."* I assume this came from me switching sides. Family would ask me how long I was planning on nursing, and I no longer had an answer. I still don't.

Shortly after Bella turned 2, I became pregnant with my second daughter, Roxanna, and my nursing relationship with Bella evolved again. At that point, I was a very active member of my local LLL group, and I took out a book from the library, *Adventures in Tandem Nursing* by Hilary Flower. I didn't know what was going to happen throughout the pregnancy. Would I be too uncomfortable to continue? Would my supply dwindle so much that Bella would lose interest?

Bella didn't lose interest, but there were definitely times when nursing was uncomfortable. I decided that I wasn't going to outright wean her but that I would be honest if I was uncomfortable. I didn't want to cringe and bear it because I was worried about damage to our relationship if I became resentful.

I thought all was well with this plan until one fateful day. I was explaining to Bella that she was going to the dentist for the first time (just like Mama and Papa) because she was a big girl with a lot of teeth. She burst into tears and cried, *"Am I being sent to the doctor because I hurt 'sides'?!"* Talk about heartbreaking! I then had to explain to her that having the baby in my tummy meant that *"sides"* hurt sometimes, and it had nothing to do with her.

She nursed all throughout the pregnancy without weaning. There was one week when she went four days without asking, and I wondered if that was the end, but no, it was not. I concluded that this was fine, and it would be a nice way to bond with her when the baby came should she have any feelings of jealousy.

Once the baby was born, my nursing relationship with Bella entered a new stage, and with it, there were new challenges. Roxy was born at home at 41 weeks; she was a good size at 7 pounds 2 ounces. There were no issues at all with breastfeeding, but of course I had a healthy baby and, at that point, was an LLL Leader. In fact, I was passing on tips to my student midwife and ended up taking a call from a struggling new mother who was a client of my midwives.

I forgot how time-consuming it was to nurse a newborn! After Roxy was a few days old and the mature milk came in, Bella latched on for the first time. She stumbled off me almost drunkenly and exclaimed, *"So much milk!"* Her patience during the pregnancy had apparently paid off.

My patience, on the other hand, was wearing a bit thin. The constant demands of nursing a newborn was taking its toll, and when Roxy wasn't nursing, I wanted to be doing anything else. Also, Bella suddenly seemed huge to me, not like a baby at all. On the plus side, any issues of engorgement that I had were quickly and easily resolved as I had the most efficient pump in the world at my house. My midwives and I joked that we would rent her out to boost supply and correct other nursing issues.

Now, Roxy is almost 11 months old, and Bella is nearly 4. I have moved from the goal of getting to 15 months to planning on letting them both self-wean. Clearly, this wasn't the plan from day 1 with Bella. It just happened one day at a time.

I realized at some point, maybe around age 2, that breastfeeding doesn't work under strict set parameters, and it still worked for all that ailed Bella, including adjusting to her new baby sister. This experience has encouraged me to allow Bella to self-wean and to aim to do the same with her sister. I don't know when either nursing relationship will end, but it seems like it will be gradual and natural, something I strive for in all aspects of parenthood (when I have the patience).

At times, it's a wonderful experience, and at times, it's utterly exhausting, like anything else in life. I still set limitations on Bella's nursing, and once Roxy is a little older, I imagine I will set limitations with her too. Bella insists that when she's 4, she will be too old to nurse. I don't think she knows how quickly 4 is coming (two months from now), and I seriously doubt that she will be done with sides.

So, the adventure continues!

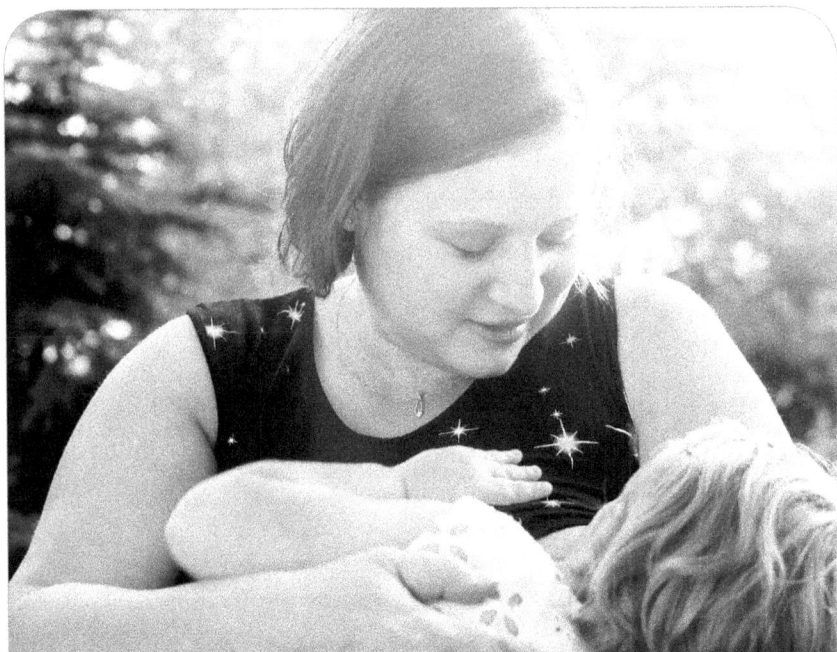

Roberta and Isabella at a nursing photo session in
June 2013 with Four Bees Photography.

Seven and Five

Lourdes M. Santaballa, Dorado, Puerto Rico

You don't plan this. Certainly when the first is born, I think that there are few who say, *"I want to do this for another seven years."* Almost two years later, when the second comes along, you don't fantasize, *"I want to continue doing this with both of them for at least another five."*

A high-need infant who nurses as often as every 20 minutes falls in love with her mother's breast. Years later, you discover it wasn't high need after all because you fulfilled all of her needs, and it was undiagnosed tongue and lip tie, but you stick it out. *"Teta"* (Spanish for breast) cures everything: hunger, hiccups, injury, loneliness, boredom, teething, growing pains, and on and on. It is the undeniable bond between you and her.

It is so strong that when 11 months later, you find out that you are pregnant, when 60% of babies supposedly wean (they say spontaneously—I think it is more often mother-initiated, but who can blame them?), she cuts back a little bit, but she is still there, no surrender. Her just reward comes nine months later, with the birth of her brother and the sweet, fatty milk that makes her drunk again.

There is that little baby, whom you cradle on the boppy; he is calm and nurses leisurely. At 20 months, she is a bit more insistent, and for six weeks, she wakes up at 5 a.m. and nurses more than her brother. You make her maneuver a bit more for it, and you give him priority, but your heart grows and your supply grows. After all, you have two tetas, not just one. The bond between you and her, you and him, is also between the three of you: where sometimes you do it one-on-one, and sometimes, they reach out and touch each other across your chest.

Time seems to pass so quickly that it is an eternity. For two-and-a-half years with him, you are still nursing five to six times a day, maybe eight times between the two of them, but weaning is a process. You start to work, there is Head Start and school, and nursing is reduced to three times a day, sometimes more on the weekends. What you could once squirt becomes droplets, but they tell you that it is sweet, that there is still milk.

There is the day at the social security office; they are 5 and 3, and they insist on public nursing. You always demand-fed. You remember that the embarrassment is yours, not theirs, and you latch them on, act like it is perfectly normal, and pretend that no one is staring at you and that maybe those who are think that it is awesome.

You make jokes that you do not nurse on demand anymore, and this is true. One of them says, *"Quiero teta" ("I want the breast"),* and you respond, *"No,"* or *"Ahora no" ("Not now"),* but sometimes you cave, and you remember the rule of giving it to them whenever food would be appropriate.

If you were Pavlov and they were the dogs, you fail on the consistency scale; they will never wean. You squeeze, and there are no droplets anymore, but they tell you that it is sweet and that there is still milk.

There is the day when she is 6 and you are at her school, and her brother insists on teta. The children ask incredulously, *"Do you still give him your milk?"*

She smiles and says, *"I still drink teta."* You ask them if any still drink a bottle sometimes. Some say yes, others gave it up last year, and others have a goal of quitting at 7. They get it. The children get it. It's the adults who have the hang-ups.

You dream about weaning. It is a be-careful-what-you-wish-for dream. When you gently nudge them to wean and talk to them about quitting, one of them tells you the next day, *"Mama, you hurt my feelings last night."*

You ask them if there is milk and you hear weaning milk is salty, but they tell you that it is sweet, and you think that this will never end. You want it to end sometimes, but there are still those sweet faces in the morning when you lie between them, and they take two sides.

This month, I've been trying more. It's been seven-and-a-half years nonstop and five-and-a-half tandem. On the weekends, I ignore them for a while and see if they fall asleep before they remember to nurse. I wake up before they do and don't offer the teta if they get up after me, and I don't wake them.

In December, I had a record of 36 hours without nursing: don't offer, don't refuse. Well, yes, I refuse sometimes. It's okay if you're nice (even if you're a little firm), and don't let anyone tell you otherwise. It's October, and I made it to 60 hours this week. I am being more conscious about it. We still cosleep. It's just the three of us now, so it's harder to get my body back, but I have that right. When I ovulate, my nipples hurt. A friend says that means that my body is telling me to wean, but weaning is a slow process if you do it the way I'm doing it. I want it to be more mother-initiated, but I don't have the heart to just take it away from them.

There was a time that I saw a 2-year-old go to his mother's lap, pull down her shirt, and latch on. It shocked me just because I had never seen it before, but it seemed okay to me. I didn't think that I'd become her or a mother with two on my lap. I remember those women I encountered at support groups or La Leche League tables, who nursed until their children were 8 or 9 and whom I thought were untouchable, and it seems like I am about to go where few go.

It's not lonely here, but we are special. It makes us closer as a trio. The children can articulate what we have. I could do standup about this or write a tear jerker, but in the end, it is just us, living an ordinary life. The days passed, and this is where we are now. Maybe she and I will make it to 8, or she'll quit, and he will continue. I don't think that it will be forever. My next goal is 72 hours. One day at a time.

The Wonders of Tandem Nursing
Olivia Hinebaugh, Burke, Virginia

Like many mothers of older nurslings, I did not set out to nurse for over three years, and I certainly did not see myself nursing through a pregnancy and birth and with a newborn. Yet, here I sit, three months after my daughter was born, still nursing with the help of my 3-year-old son, and I am so happy that it worked out this way.

I half expected my son Callum to wean during pregnancy. I read all about how the milk supply dwindles and turns into weaning milk, which is saltier. He even told me that my milk tasted different. He's a passionate nurser, and none of this dissuaded him—not even when my milk dried up completely after the first trimester.

My breasts were sore. Every time he latched on, I had to fight the urge to grimace. Nursing him to sleep was exhausting me. He needed the breast in his mouth to soothe him to sleep, and my attempts to extract my nipple from between his teeth and his lazy latch would often wake him up. Tired from pregnancy, I often just gave up and, still nursing, fell asleep next to him.

As the months wore on and my belly made fitting into bed with him difficult, I made the tough choice to night-wean him. It was a tough time for me, but the amount that we were nursing was wearing me out. I experienced a lot of guilt from taking that comfort away from him. I hated to hear his tears. I struggled to stay in my room and let my husband deal with his tantrums. It only took a few nights of explaining that my breasts were tired for him to learn to just snuggle to sleep. A large part of me was ready to wean altogether. I wasn't sure that I was tough enough to nurse two babies, but another part of me wanted to just wait and see what would happen.

Callum continued to nurse in the daytime. He looked forward to the morning when I would agree that the sun was out and that he could resume nursing when he asked. I could still nurse him if he was hurt or upset, and there was a perk that I had taken for granted until I was exhausted in my third trimester: nursing allowed us to slow down and rest in the middle of the day.

Callum gave up napping around the time that I got pregnant, but I could still coax him to lie down and snuggle with me to read a book or nurse. This realization made me glad that he was still an enthusiastic nursling.

Any mother of two or more children can relate to the worries I had as the birth approached. My baby, the center of my world, was no longer going to be an only child. He was going to have to share me and my husband with a newer, needier child. I knew I would cope. My own mother reassured me that I would have room in my heart for both children, but I wasn't entirely convinced.

When I awoke in early labor on the day of my daughter's birth, my first thought was of Callum. I was excited and eager, of course. I buzzed around the house, preparing for our home birth and excitedly calling my midwife. When labor got a little more serious and my contractions were only a few minutes apart, I knew that I wanted to savor my beautiful little boy's last day as my baby. I invited him into my room to nurse. He climbed onto my perfectly made bed, lay down beside me, and curled his legs around my large belly as he had learned to do. It was blissful. I know that my body was surging with birth hormones that intensified this moment, but it was pure magic. My contractions grew much more intense at his suckling, and I told him that he was actually helping me to open up and make room for his baby sister to come out. He smiled and nodded. He knew all about this. It had been the main topic of conversation in the previous weeks when he demanded, *"Mom, can you push the baby out now?"*

I told him that we had to be patient. The door to my womb had to open first. He was excited, and so was I. We had also discussed how he could help me when I was working hard through labor. When I told him that I was having a contraction, he reached up and rubbed my forehead, and I couldn't stop kissing his blonde curls. My husband was in the room and took pictures. I treasure these pictures.

His nursing really did kick my labor into a higher gear. Things got serious, and soon, my midwife arrived and told me I was already dilated 7 centimeters. Callum came in my room a few more times to rub my back or put ice on my head. He was so sweet. We didn't nurse any more until after his sister Lucy was born.

He came in shortly after her birth. He wanted to see the cord, so we waited to cut it. When he entered the room, he marveled at her and watched as the cord was cut. I put Lucy back to my breast. I held my breath, unsure of how Callum would react. We had discussed that this was what babies did a lot of the time, but it was different in practice than in reality.

"She's nursing?" he asked me.

"Yes, she is."

"Can I nurse?" he asked.

So, he snuggled under my arm and nursed on the other breast. Callum was very contented. He couldn't keep his eyes off of Lucy. In a gesture of pure adoration, he reached across my chest and took Lucy's tiny hand in his.

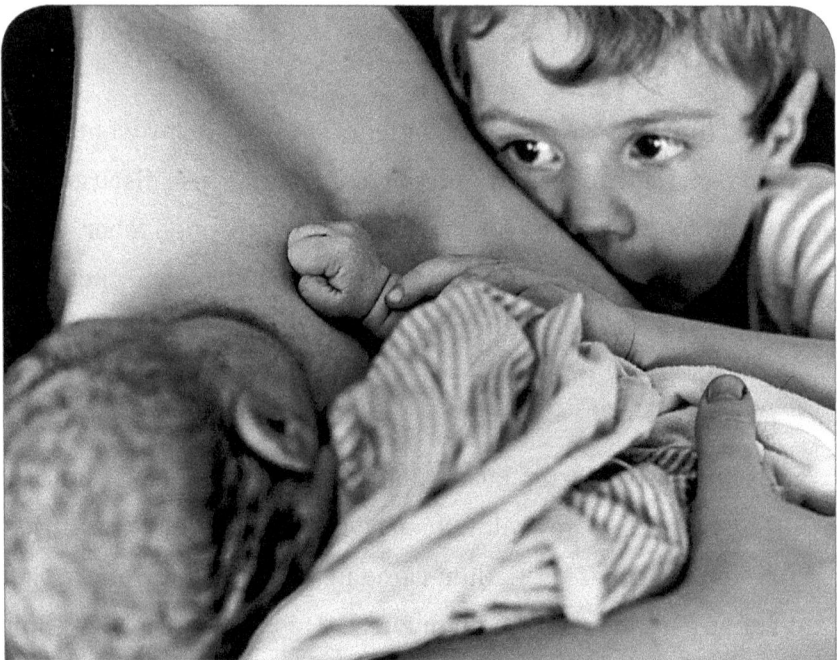

Tandem nursing helped Olivia's children bond. Here, her son looked over at Olivia's newborn daughter and took her hand.

Callum loves his little sister. In those first few weeks, he acted out a bit at his diminished attention, but he is only ever completely loving with Lucy. He often joins in when I'm feeding Lucy. I think in a lot of ways that the continuation of our nursing relationship prevented jealousy. He needed nursing more than ever. It was an easy way for me to show him that I still cared and would still nurture him.

Now that Lucy is 3 months old, they still nurse together occasionally, and Callum will still hold her hand. I couldn't have asked for a better start to Callum's role as a big brother. I still find it amazing and beautiful that his nursing helped my labor progress quickly and that, in his way, he helped welcome the newest member of our family.

Nursing through pregnancy was certainly not easy, but I can say with confidence that it was worth it. It was worth it for that last moment with him as my baby, and it was worth it to have two contented nurslings in our house. I was hopeful that it could be this way, but it was better than I even imagined.

Balancing Needs and Chances
Marti, United Kingdom

Before I ever got pregnant with my first child, I imagined that I would get pregnant again within a year after birth. I was almost 30 and planning to have at least four children well before I turned 40. I never thought that I would be one of those women struggling to conceive. I was wrong.

Eventually, I had my first baby. They say that breastfeeding doesn't protect against conception after six months, and I took this to mean that after six months, my fertility would be back. How wrong I was! I didn't get my periods back until my daughter was 1, and even then, my luteal phase was too short to sustain a pregnancy. How jealous I was of all of the mothers complaining that their periods came back soon after birth! By the time my daughter was 2, I was desperately broody. I was past caring about how my new baby would be born, how he or she would be fed, even whether he or she would be healthy! I just wanted a baby!

At that time, I seriously considered weaning my daughter. While I'd considered weaning several times before (and after), I was never as serious about it. I needed a baby, and breastfeeding was an obstacle in my way. What a dilemma! Should I wean and maybe fail to conceive anyway? It would feel like failing my child, a child who did not come easily and who was not ready to wean. Should I continue to breastfeed and perhaps give up the chance of having another baby? Would the broody feeling ever go away? Would I end up resenting my child for being so needy? I was starting to accept the idea that

I would not be able to have the four children that I wanted, but the idea of having only one child was unthinkable!

Just as I was referred to the fertility clinic, I got pregnant, and the reason to wean my daughter was no longer there, so we continued.

I didn't experience any problems in pregnancy. My daughter was sleeping in her own room and had milk mornings and evenings, sometimes only once, and sometimes not at all. I was wondering if she would wean, but she continued.

Then, her brother was born a month after her third birthday, and she was jealous of the attention he was getting. When he was having milk, she wanted some milk too. She wanted milk when he was sleeping. All she wanted was milk. I guess for her it was a symbol of mummy's love. How could I deny her?

Many tandem-feeding mums are familiar with *"the irritation,"* otherwise known as *nursing aversion.* I had none in pregnancy, but it hit after birth. It's difficult to describe what it's like. It's very primal. It's a very strong urge to remove the older nursling from the breast *now:* push them, punch them, whatever! I wonder if animals feel the same when they kick their young away or get up and run off?! Obviously, being human and having the capacity for rational thought, I never gave in to this urge, but I had to find a way to make nursing more bearable. Limiting the amount of feeds was not a viable option, so I tried limiting the duration while being respectful of my daughter and not making her feel rejected. I came up with a game: she could choose a short song, and I would sing it while she nursed. When the song was over, she had to stop. Then, she needed to think of another song. She could have several songs; the pauses between were just long enough to make it bearable for me. The first few months were overwhelming.

It gradually passed. I don't remember when I stopped feeling irritated. I don't remember when my daughter cut down to one to two feeds per day. It just happened very gradually. When my son was around 1, he became very jealous. I had to stop feeding them at the same time then because he would hurt his sister. Now that he is 2, I can sometimes feed them both. I just lie on my back in bed and let them get on with it, and they can usually do it without fighting. They fight all day, so it's nice to have a peaceful morning at least.

When my daughter was born, I didn't quite know how to be a mother. I'm still learning. I fed her on a schedule and tried to avoid feeding her to sleep. She also had formula sometimes to *"get her used to it."* I tried making my husband give her a bottle at 10 p.m. so that I could get some sleep (I always woke up anyway). I just thought that was the way to do it. I didn't feed her in public after the first eight or so months (partly because I was self-conscious and partly because she wanted both breasts out at the same time). I went back to work part-time when she was 9 months old, and she had formula in daycare. We coslept from about 4 months to over 2 years (we only had one bedroom, so it was partly out of necessity). We night-weaned her when she was 2 by moving her over to Daddy's side. She was used to Daddy doing bedtimes, so she didn't expect milk from him. If she slept on my side, she would still wake for milk. Also, when she was 2½, we moved, and she got her own bedroom.

I am a lot more relaxed about breastfeeding my son. I've learned a lot more about parenting and a lot more about breastfeeding too. I became self-employed, so he's not had much daycare either. We tried, but he cried when I left him, and I felt guilty, so I pulled him out as soon as it was possible. While my daughter slept in a Moses basket initially, my son was in a bedside cot from the beginning, and he is still there now at 28 months old. He is mostly breastfed to sleep. He never took a bottle. He wakes in the night, and I'm not fussy about night weaning. I feel reassured that I can limit his daytime feeds if needed, as he can wake up in the night and get all the milk that he needs. He will have to share a bedroom with his sister at some point, but I don't want to move him before he is night-weaned because I don't want him waking her up. I also don't want him waking up everybody early in the morning. If he is right next to me, he can have milk and go back to sleep or at least doze on and off.

I am 36 now. Have I given up on my plan of having four children? I don't know. I would maybe like another baby at some point, but at the moment, it is more important that I meet the needs of the children I already have, and this includes breastfeeding them until they decide it's time to wean, even if it is affecting my fertility. Sometimes, I even consider the option of not having any more children, and sometimes I think that's okay.

From Formula Mum to Lactivist

Sharon Spink, Sherburn in Elmet, North Yorkshire, England

When Charlotte was born in 2009, I was so determined to breastfeed successfully that I don't think anything or anyone would or could have stopped me. Having had what I thought of as three failed attempts to breastfeed, I knew that this time I had to have as much support and information as possible. I knew she was going to be another cesarean section baby, but because I had done it three times before, that wasn't a worry. What I was worried about was getting breastfeeding started as soon as possible. I knew all about how important it was to feed within the first hour after birth. I needn't have worried.

We got off to a great start, but like any breastfeeding mum, I came up against problems: sore nipples, growth spurts where she would want to feed almost constantly for 12 to 15 hours at a time for a couple of days at a time, occasional negative comments, biting while feeding, thrush, and my trying to start a new business.

Well, the weeks and months flew by, and soon Charlotte was 6 months old, then 12 months old. Before I knew it, she was a walking, talking toddler who was happily asking for *"mummy milk,"* although she had been signing for milk from about 8 months. Trying to breastfeed with an older child around was much easier than I thought, definitely easier than if I had been having to prepare bottles. My older daughter Isabel was at nursery a couple of mornings a week, so Charlotte and I had our one-on-one time together. My husband was also great. When it was just me and the two younger kids, I would find things to keep Isabel happy while I fed Charlotte, or we would just sit cuddling on the sofa watching television or reading a book. Isabel was very intrigued by how I was feeding Charlotte, even asking if she could have a go. I let her, but she changed her mind at the last second and ran off giggling. I would often find Isabel copying me by breastfeeding her dolls. It was lovely to see that she was growing up seeing breastfeeding as the normal way to feed babies and children.

As time went on, I realized that I was slowly becoming a bit of a lactivist. I joined several breastfeeding-related groups on Facebook, and after seeing a group organize a flash mob in London, I decided to organize my own in Leeds to coincide with National Breastfeeding Awareness Week and to help promote breastfeeding in public. I think that I managed to get about 40 mums to join me in the middle of Leeds City Station. We caused quite a stir, but apart from a couple of negative comments, it was a very positive way of promoting breastfeeding.

When in 2012, Jamie Lynne Grumet was shown on the front of *Time* magazine breastfeeding her almost 4-year-old, it was amazing. At last, someone had shown the world that it was normal. Unfortunately, the strap line of *"Are You Mom Enough?"* did us no favors. You don't need to be a certain type of mum to be an extended breastfeeder. We're just mums. As a result of this article, ITV's *This Morning* contacted the Association of Breastfeeding Mothers and asked to interview a mum of an older breastfed child. I responded to that and ended up appearing on the show while breastfeeding Charlotte, who was 3 at the time. I then had an interview to discuss why I was breastfeeding an older child and put my point across in a very calm and knowledgeable way. I showed my nation that breastfeeding a toddler is perfectly normal. I did receive a lot of negative comments from viewers, but I definitely don't regret doing the interview and would happily do it again. The support that I got from the breastfeeding community was unbelievable. I felt very proud to be the face of long-term breastfeeding mums for that small moment in time.

Breastfeeding a toddler or preschooler has its own challenges. They are much bigger, for instance, so sometimes finding a suitable chair in restaurants and other public places can be a struggle. They love to try out different positions too: *"Ooh, will my leg go up there and my arm down there? What if I twist round here? Can I watch television while feeding?"* However, it also has its rewards. Charlotte loves to hug and kiss my breasts and tell me she loves them. She also tells me that one side tastes of ice cream and the other side tastes of chocolate, but that can vary.

We live in a small village, and I'm certainly the exception to the rule. I don't know anyone else here who is breastfeeding a toddler let alone a school-aged child. I have one or two friends that wear their babies with a wrap or Mei Tei carrier but none who have breastfed long term. My friends accept that I follow my instincts with my parenting style when it comes to breastfeeding and raising my children, but I have learned not to shove it down their throats too. We all have different parenting styles, and we respect one other and our choices.

Charlotte and I have a lovely breastfeeding relationship, and it doesn't matter where we are. If Charlotte needs feeding, then I feed her. She even came with me to my grandpa's funeral, just in case she needed the comfort of mummy milk. She didn't, although I got lots of comfort from her being there. I have had a few comments from some family members about when I am going to stop breastfeeding, but the answer that they get is always the same: *"When Charlotte is ready to stop!"* She loves to breastfeed, so why would I want to take that away from her?

Charlotte started full-time school in September 2013, and it hasn't affected her breastfeeding other than the fact that she can now feed only most mornings and at bedtime. If we're together all day, then there will be times when she still asks for mummy milk. She doesn't mind where we are; breastfeeding is just normal to her. It's our morning cuddles, her comfort when she's upset, her way of reconnecting with me when we've been apart, and her bedtime drink to help her settle before going to sleep. I'm not looking forward to the day when she finally stops breastfeeding, but I really didn't think we'd be going for this long, so I am very proud of our breastfeeding journey. Long may it continue!

A Natural Progression
Lorah Smith, California

I have three children, but before I had any, I knew that I would breastfeed them. I simply wanted to because it seemed like the best, most healthy option. I, of course, had no idea of the challenges, obstacles, or joy that it would bring. When my son was born, my goal was a year. I'm not sure why that was my goal back then, but it seemed like a good one. I didn't know how hard it would be or how it would work, but once we started, I quickly adapted! I was all about the amazing life of a breastfeeding mama. I would nurse on request, no matter the time of day or where we were. He hated covers, so I adjusted to nursing how he wanted and grew confident with nursing in public, albeit still modestly, but I never shied away or hid. So, when he self-weaned at 15 months, I literally sobbed for a week. I'm so very glad that his weaning is not the end of my story.

Six months after my son weaned, I conceived my second child, a daughter. This time, the plan was to encourage breastfeeding for at least two years, as the more I read, the more that's what made sense for development, health, and attachment. I knew that since I practiced child-led weaning, my goal of two years might not happen, especially since my first weaned young, but from the moment she was born, I had a feeling that we were destined to have a long-lasting breastfeeding relationship!

The second my daughter was born, she rooted and inched toward my breast, and within hours of her birth, she was a champion nurser! The midwife was amazed at how well we were both doing. I have to say that I felt blessed to have things going so smoothly for both my daughter and me from the start. Basically, from that moment on, she was nearly always attached, and we both loved it!

When she hit 2 years, she was still nursing around the clock, and I was so very excited that we had reached my desired two-year mark. Each and every second after her second birthday I counted as a gift. When people asked me if she was still breastfeeding, I would just say yes and that I doubted she would be going off to college still asking for *"mommy milk"* or *"boobie snacks,"* and we went about our lives happily. We went to nurse-ins together, celebrated World Breastfeeding Day a few years, and even participated in the world record for simultaneous breastfeeding mamas and nurslings. Really, it was just part of life. It wasn't anything out of the ordinary for us, and I guess that she just projected a sense of confidence because, thankfully, no one ever approached us to object.

Shortly after she turned 2, I realized that although I loved our cuddles and our nursing time together, my body was wearing out. I simply was not getting enough sleep, as she was continuing to wake every 2 hours to nurse. Although I very strongly believe in child-led weaning, I also knew that we both needed more sleep, so I developed my own gentle, no-cry, child-assisted method for night weaning. I decided to alternate nursing with rocking and singing. At her first waking, I would nurse her. At her second waking, I would rock and sing to her, and at the third waking, I would nurse her. I did this for as long as it took for her to eventually just sleep through those rocking-and-singing wakings. Then, I'd wait a week, and start alternating the remaining wakings. I did this until we were finally down to one waking per night. Then, we had a talk about how the mommy milk would be full during the day, but at night, it needed to fill back up while we both got some sleep. Then, as the sun went down that first night, we nursed. She went to bed with songs I sang to her. When she woke, I held her and told her I loved her, and she went peacefully back to sleep. It took a couple of months altogether, but we were finally sleeping, and I was still being greeted at the crack of dawn for nursing and snuggles. It was amazing.

We had made it to 2 1/2 years! We were both happy, sleeping, and nursing, and I thought life was perfect! Then, I started to get mastitis: not once, not twice, but many, many times. I never understood why women would give up breastfeeding over an infection until I started to get them. I had a new sense of empathy and understanding. I also was more determined than ever to push through it. I thought to myself, *"I've made it this far. I'm not giving up without a fight."* After a few months, I found a groove and learned that certain positions were not as good as others, and we were good. I felt like if I could make it through that, I could make it through anything.

Two months after her third birthday, I conceived my third child. I had a few people expecting me to wean. Some told me to wean, but nope, I knew my body could do it, and so we kept at it. Despite the discomfort in the first trimester, including sore nipples and bruised ducts, we still very much enjoyed our snuggling and nursing time together. In my second trimester, she would comment on the taste change or quantity change, but we both were still happy with our morning cuddles and mommy milk time. We talked about how she would share with the baby. She would even say, *"I'll let the baby go first. Then, I'll have some too."* Sure enough, when the baby was born, although they never simultaneously tandem-nursed (much to my dismay), she always let her baby sister go first and would smile, sit close, and snuggle with us, all the while talking to the baby and telling her how good the milk was and how she was happy to share.

In the months to follow, she watched as the baby would nurse, and she would ask for milk every so often, but I could see the natural progression of things that was leading her to be more of a big sister and less of a baby. She would encourage the baby to nurse, telling the baby how good it was, and sometimes latch for a moment, but ultimately, it seemed to be more for demonstration. A few days after her fourth birthday, she asked for mommy milk for the last time. I knew it was the last time because she had been spacing out her nursings for a while by then, and this time she asked for it in a cup. She took a few sips, looked at me, smiled, and said, *"Mommy, I'm a big girl now. I will let my baby sister have the mommy milk now,"* and that was that. My heart was not crushed as I had thought it would be like when my son weaned, but it was not happy either. I did feel contented and proud though. I was proud that we were able to have such a wonderful four years. I feel blessed to have been able to offer her the ability to have the experience for as long as she wanted.

I am still breastfeeding the baby, although I should probably start calling her a kid, as she is over a year old, is running and climbing, and is anything but a baby. I hope to allow her to breastfeed as long as she wishes, be it 15 months, four years, or whenever the end organically presents itself.

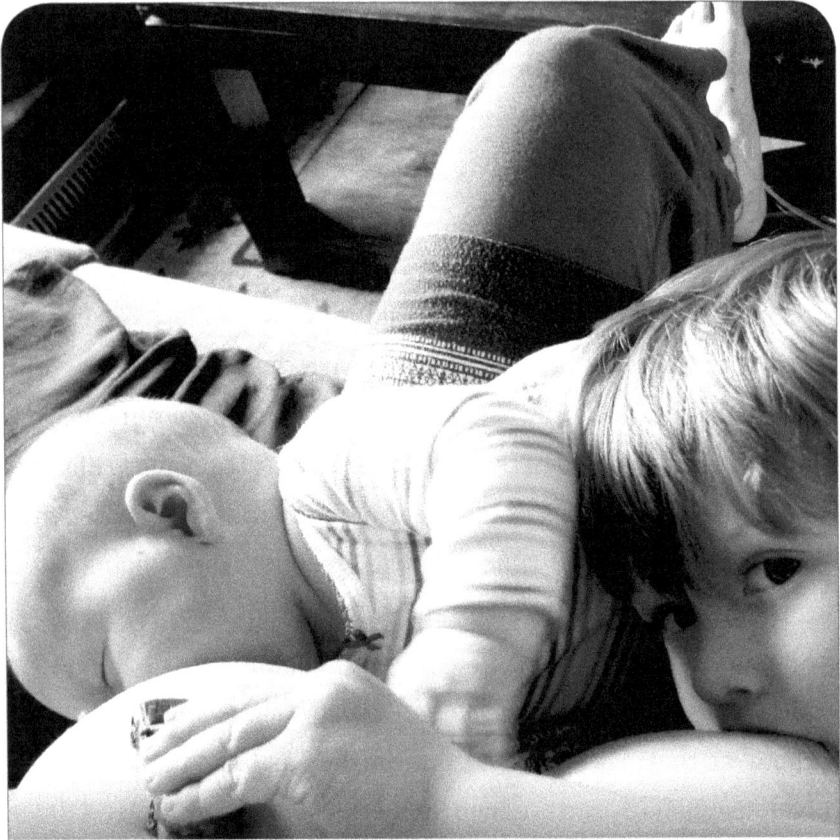

Pauline Osborne, Redmond, Washington, tandem-nursing her 4-month-old daughter and her 3½-year-old son, who loves playing with his cars while he nurses.

Continuing by Setting Limits
Vicky, Norwich, England

My son Eddie is only three months away from his fourth birthday, and we're still breastfeeding. I had a little think and calculated roughly in my head the other day that I must have fed him at least 4000 times. I've never calculated how many times I've kissed, cuddled, or told him that I love him, but those things are unconditional and unlimited. Breastfeeding has not been, not always. As much as it pained me, sometimes I had to set some limits.

Ed was born at 12:45 a.m. on a Sunday morning after three days of never really getting into established labor. His heart trace was never satisfactory, and the contractions never really got going until, exhausted and frightened, I gave in and let them do whatever the hell they wanted to just get him out. That meant an epidural, syntocin drip, and constant attachment to a monitor. After his heart rate suddenly dropped for the second time, they decided it was time for an emergency C-section. A terrified me rang my mother in tears—the whole experience had been the complete opposite of what I had wanted—before I was wheeled off to be sliced up.

He came out blue and not moving. I apparently giggled my head off as they stitched me up and revived him. I was numb from the neck down, so I couldn't even hold my boy until he was about 6 hours old. There went the immediate skin-to-skin contact. My husband was sent home as Ed had been born in the middle of the night, and I was left alone with this fascinating little being, whom I instinctively wanted close to me but had no way to physically hold.

No one suggested that I attempt to feed him, and he was asleep, so I didn't think to try. When we finally got around to it, he wouldn't latch. Any number of midwives and maternity care assistants tried to shove my boob in his mouth, but he just wouldn't do it, so I hand-expressed and fed him with a syringe. I was like a pro apparently. I got 20 milliliters of colostrum, and this was then held up and shown off to all the other new mothers on the ward. I bet that made them feel great!

Eventually, someone gave me a nipple shield to try, and it just worked. Well, he stayed on and fed at any rate. That second night of his existence in the world was just a blur of tears (his and mine), sterilizing, and snatched minutes of sleep. He was feeding but never seemed satisfied.

When I got pregnant, I was determined to breastfeed. My husband wanted to get some formula and bottles *"just in case,"* but I refused. I remember reading my notes in the hospital, and the thing that stuck out was the phrase *"failure to progress"* as the reason for my emergency C-section. Wow. That made me feel like the worst mother in the world and also made me even more determined not to fail to feed him as I had failed to birth him.

So, I got sent home. I could feed him only in the rugby ball hold thanks to my C-section wound. It took a carefully balanced pile of cushions to get in a semicomfortable position. I had to keep cleaning and sterilizing the nipple shield. I'm not going to lie: I did not enjoy it one bit, except for having the opportunity to look down into the beautiful face of my happy little boy. He didn't mind.

My midwife told me the reason that he couldn't latch on was that my nipples were too small and that the nipple shields were working, so I should carry on. My health visitor told me that I risked diminishing my supply if I didn't stop using them but offered no advice on how to stop.

Three weeks later, I was getting to the limit of how much I could endure. I remember crying, not for the first time, to my mum that breastfeeding was supposed to be magic. I did not feel the magic. Luckily for me, my mum had a friend who was a breastfeeding counselor. She dropped everything to come and help me. She reassured me that my nipples were perfectly adequate and really gave me the confidence to persevere. Just three days later, Ed himself decided he was not going to feed with the nipple shields, and I threw the damn things in the bin! I felt the magic after that most of the time.

He was never a *"good"* sleeper. We were permanently exhausted for the first year of his life. At 14 months, I knew that it was time for night weaning. Luckily for me, I have a very supportive mum who has a great bond with Eddie. I went to stay at mum's for a week while my husband was away for work. I was downstairs in case I was needed, but Ed was upstairs with mum, who was armed with expressed breast milk in a beaker and Nana's soothing touch.

It wasn't easy. He cried. He refused the breast milk. I wondered if I was doing the right thing. Then, by the fourth night, he just got it. He still woke up, but he settled very quickly with a cuddle and a back rub from Nana. Looking back, I feel a little uncomfortable. I have never, ever done controlled crying, and I know that this was different as he always had the support of someone who loved him, someone he trusted, but I'd never denied him a feed before.

After that, my husband co-slept with Eddie. That way, there was someone there if he woke, but he didn't expect me or milk. A part of me felt like I should have been there for him, but it was a lovely way for him and his daddy to bond, and they still are very close.

As Ed's second birthday approached, I was still feeding him several times a day and, much to the horror of many friends, feeding him to sleep at night. I was starting to enjoy it less. He has always been a big boy, and feeding was no longer a gentle, cuddly experience. He had this habit of shoving his free hand up my sleeve and scratching and picking my arm while feeding. It drove me insane! I could find nothing to stop him. I started to try the old *"never sit down"* trick so that he couldn't climb on my lap and ask for a feed, but I always had to give in at some point.

It made me feel awful as I wanted him to decide when to stop, but I was getting to a point where feeding was irritating, not magic. Then, his daddy had two weeks off work. Like magic, Ed seemed to forget about breastfeeding during the day. Playing with Daddy was just so much fun! He would crawl into bed with me for a half-awake feed in the morning, and we carried on feeding to sleep but with nothing in between.

I was greatly relieved, although not without some doubts and some guilt. I remembered a discussion from baby group when our little ones turned 1. Everyone was talking about their children's security blankets and favorite toys that they couldn't be without. I said that Eddie had never had such an object. One of my friends exclaimed, *"Of course not! He uses you!"* I know that she meant it in a less than positive way, but she was right, and it made me feel proud. I always kept this in mind when deciding whether to feed Ed during the day. There was no blanket ban, but rather I'd judge his mood and whether he really needed the comfort or whether he was just bored and could be entertained with something else.

As his third birthday got closer, I felt the need to stop the morning feeds. He was starting nursery, school, and hour-long feeds in the morning just meant such a rush to get ready and out the door, so I started using a little trick that still works for almost everything: setting a timer. I'd set my phone alarm for 10 minutes, and when it went off, he got to press the button to stop it! Being allowed to touch my phone was so exciting that he did not fuss about the feed ending.

So now, with him 4 years old, we just have the one feed at night to get him to sleep. It works most of the time; other times, he just gets in bed and goes to sleep. These haven't been extreme limits, and I've relaxed them at times, like when he has been ill and refusing all other sustenance. I sometimes wonder when (if?) we'll stop, but every night when I cuddle up to my beautiful son, tell him I love him, and watch his peaceful little face as he suckles himself to sleep, I hope that it's not for a while yet.

Chapter 4

Support Makes All the Difference

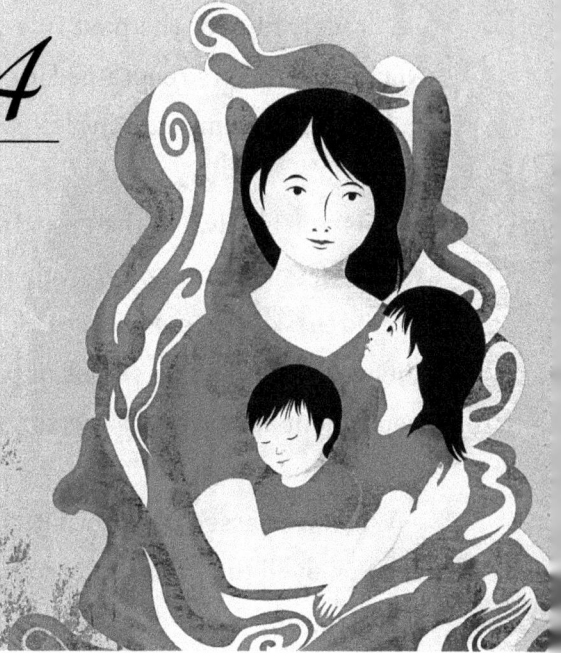

When a mother is in a nursing relationship with a small infant or child, she needs the support of the people who are close to her. Her spouse or partner and her extended family can be the very cornerstone that she needs to follow her child's cues and her own instincts and figure out what is best for them both. Without that support or, worse, with active opposition, the full-term breastfeeding journey can be difficult and strenuous at best. Fortunately, mothers can reach out to friends and support groups, such as La Leche League, to supplement their own support systems or to make up for the lack of one.

Support Within

Jessica Dee Humphreys, Canada

Tasked with writing about the breastfeeding support that I have received over the past five years, I couldn't find the words. Nursing has been so engrained in our family life that I found it almost impossible to segregate that experience.

This wasn't always the case. In the first years, I reveled in the worthiness of nursing. I actively participated in advocacy and celebrated the *"anytime, anywhere"* doctrine passionately. I delighted in the warm supportive smiles of passersby and was buoyed by the benevolent approval of experts.

When we passed the internationally sanctioned two-year mark, I then enjoyed the pride of fiercely being part of a more select movement: a group of powerful women who felt that they were listening to their own wisdom, respecting their children, and not allowing their lives to be dictated by medical professionals led by corporate lucre.

At 4 years, however, my personal role models detached (literally). I floundered, unsure, abandoned. I sought out the limited published expertise available and was again cast adrift: the two well-intentioned books that I found on nursing children over 3 were merely platforms for detailing and combatting negativity, derision, scorn, and judgment: all experiences of which I had been blissfully ignorant! With eyes so ruthlessly pried open to the reality of society's censure of my behavior, I unwillingly initiated weaning and was met with an inarguable and plaintive argument from my son: *"But I love it!"*

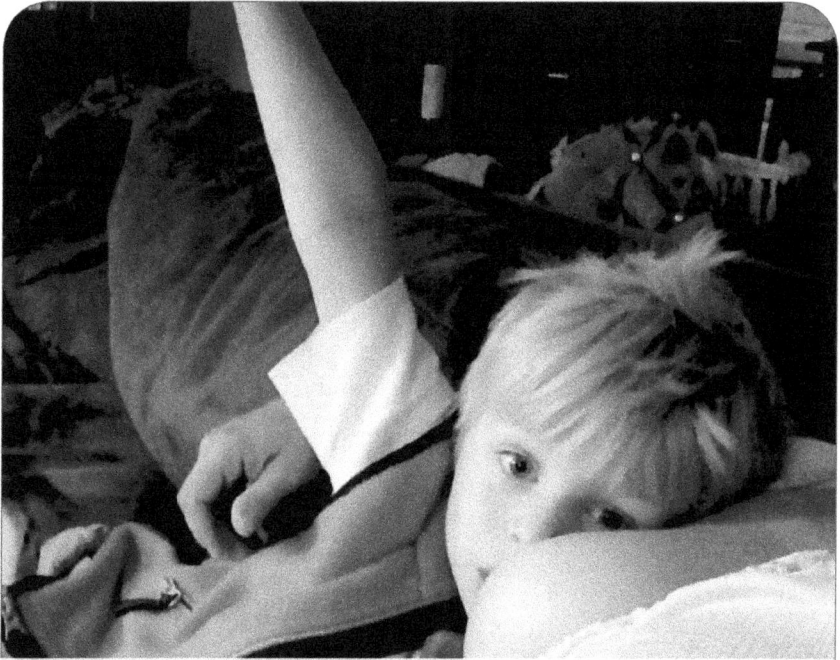

According to Jessica, nursing a 4-year-old isn't always like the gentle bonding that you had with your baby, but it is always joyful!

©2013 Jessica Dee Humphreys.

So, in the past year, we have looked only within and not without for our support. I joyfully discovered our strongest allies, who had been with us all along. Alongside my child and me, my partner and my mom have been so absolute, so silent, and so stalwart in their unwavering support that I had failed to appreciate or even notice the cornerstone that they had provided.

Nursing has thus become to us as natural, necessary, and mundane as air. The Garden of Eden was mundane too: it was beautiful, peaceful, and providing; it was the time and place for innocence, kindness, and love; and it was necessarily fleeting, ephemeral, and terminable.

When I try to capture our long-term nursing experience on paper, prose fails me, so I turn to the poetic:

> *In me You moved*
> *from ovum*
> *to arms*
>
> *embraced and fed*
> *always*
> *sweet, warm, assured.*
>
> *a true eden:*
> *Thou mayest freely eat*
> *pleasant and good.*
>
> *The Root and the fruit*
> *sucking and giving*
> *delight is sustaining*
>
> *garden of the East*
> *dawns fresh and pure*
> *innocenti.*
>
> *a Man shall leave his father and his mother*
> *and yet, so long ... so long,*
> *a Babe in arms shall rest a while*
>
> *there is time.*

One N for Soothing My Child
Sarah Diener Beachy, Fulks Run, Virginia

I have been very fortunate to have the support of my family in continuing to nurse my son Sam. He has been nursing for over four years, and the caring and love that my husband and extended family have shown toward us have encouraged me to continue toward my goal of nursing Sam until he is ready to wean.

My husband Ben joined in my commitment to breastfeed Sam before he was born. When newborn Sam woke up wet and crying in the cosleeper, Ben would change his diaper and then bring him back to me to nurse. During the first days when we were figuring out nursing, Ben helped me get arranged with our tiny squirmy baby, who seemed to be all flailing limbs and bobbing head. He cooked me breakfast while I nursed. He fetched glasses of water, another burp rag, my book, my laptop, a footstool, or whatever I needed while I sat on the couch. Ben was the one who found out what bright green diaper contents meant and how to fix it. When I felt overwhelmed, he was there with encouragement and kind words.

When Sam was a small baby, Ben helped ensure that we weren't separated. He always brought Sam to me when he needed to nurse. If I had an appointment or meeting, Ben would go along with Sam, so he could bring him to me as soon as I was available. He made countless pit stops by the side of the road for me to get Sam out of his car seat when he needed nursing. We planned times that the two of us could connect without having to leave Sam. All three of us counted on nursing as the cure-all.

Ben deferred to me on sleeping arrangements, the timing and composition of Sam's first solid foods, and other matters concerning Sam. He read the books and blogs I that suggested and supported my choices in parenting Sam. Sam had a special smile that he gave Ben whenever he came home and picked him up.

When Sam was a year old, he was still nursing for most of his nutrition. He would try a variety of foods but didn't consume them in any significant quantity until after his second birthday. Ben continued to support our nursing relationship. One night, I woke up to Ben saying, *"Wrong one,"* and gently turning Sam in my direction from where he had been questing on Ben's side of the bed.

Playfulness has always been a big part of Ben's relationship with Sam. It has for me as well, but I'm pretty sure *"giver of milk"* overshadowed *"play partner"* with me frequently!

Ben would ask Sam if he wanted to nurse on him instead, a suggestion that was always met with vehement denial, or Ben would pretend he was going to drink the milk instead of Sam. Though Sam always rejected these offers, this playfulness made Ben more of an apparent part of our nursing relationship. I think that Ben's participation in this dual activity drew us closer as a family rather than pushing him outside of this part of our family relationship.

When Sam was 3, I heard a radio interview with Harvey Karp, the author of the Happiest Baby on the Block books. I described to Ben this author's five S's for soothing a baby. Ben's comment was, *"I think one N would be simpler,"* "N" being for nursing, of course!

Ben's support and encouragement have helped me greatly during difficult phases of nursing. When Sam was nearing 4 and was still nursing several times during the night, I described to Ben a plan for night weaning that I was thinking of trying. Ben expressed surprise and reminded me that up to this point, I had always said that I would let Sam choose when and how to wean.

Ben offered to try other sleeping arrangements instead to help us all get more sleep. I rethought my plan, and we did some bed rearranging and decided to wait. Several months later, Sam was nursing only once about every other night and then easily gave it up with a gentle push from me. I am very glad that I had waited. I think that at the earlier point, it would have been nights and nights of protests and anguish.

My family has been wonderful in their support as well. My mother was a La Leche League Leader and has given me information and support, as well as stories of nursing her four children (two of us past 3 years). My brothers, sister, and their spouses don't blink an eye when I nurse Sam in front of them.

My sister remembers nursing and has told me about the warmth and closeness that she remembers feeling, and this has been a great encouragement to me in nursing Sam past his baby years.

I share a house with my parents-in-law and was unsure about how they would react to Sam continuing to nurse past age 2. They have been wonderfully kind and understanding. My mother-in-law has told me that she wishes she had had more support in nursing her children when they were babies and was very encouraging when I was working to become a La Leche League Leader myself.

Nursing a child past 4 is not something that I bring up with many of my acquaintances. Sam rarely asks when we're in social situations, and I'm sure that most people assume that we stopped nursing years ago. Some of my close friends know that Sam still nurses, and if someone asks directly, I will usually tell him because if a person thinks to ask whether a 4-year-old is still nursing, it's usually because he or she is okay with it! I am very glad that I don't feel like I have to hide from my family though.

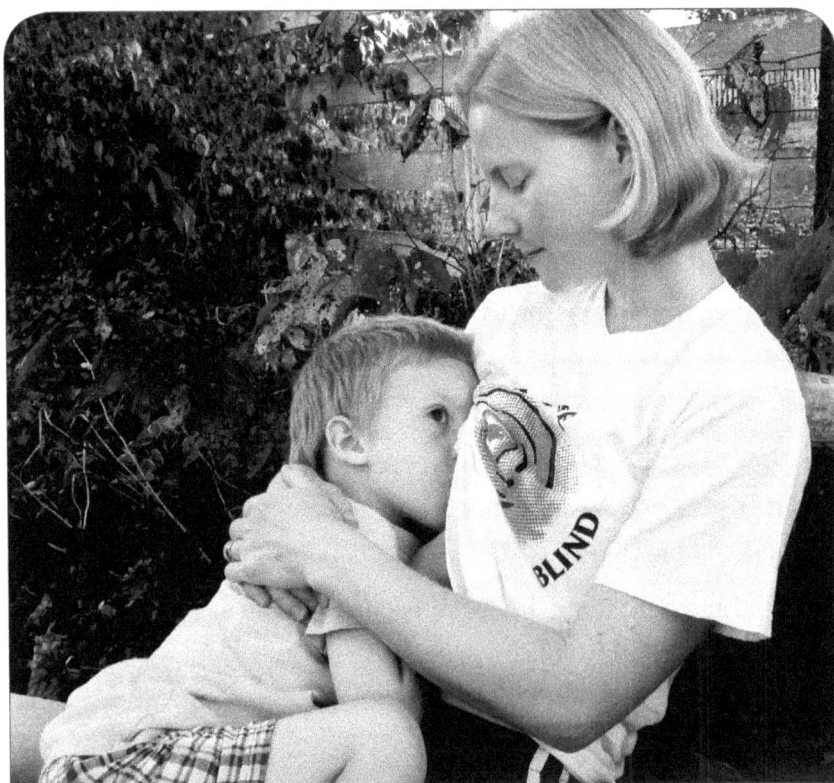

Sam, 4, enjoys an outdoor nursing break with his mother, Sarah.

Sam is now 4½ and nurses at bedtime and in the morning with occasional times in between.

At this point, nursing is pretty easy and convenient. It's a nice way to get him to sleep at night, it's handy if I need him to be quiet for a few minutes while I'm on the phone, and it still helps to soothe hurts of all kinds. At the same time, he doesn't have to nurse if it's not convenient, and he will accept alternatives.

Sometimes, it seems like he must be on his way to weaning soon. He says he will nurse until he's 6. Whatever happens, his family will be there with their love and support.

How Breastfeeding Saved My Life

Andrea Samaniego, Buenos Aires, Argentina

L ife is full of coincidences. However, I really do not believe in coincidence, but I do believe in causality.

I wanted to start with this first statement because I feel that the story I am telling was due to be written at this particular moment of my daughter's life: yes, right now, when my little daughter is about to finish with her latency. At least, that is what she seems to be trying to show me as our breastfeeding sessions are becoming shorter and shorter and she does not latch on at night any more.

Let me present myself as a mom: I was an old cow full of misconceptions about pregnancy and lactation. I was a well-organized, professional in her forties with no brothers or sisters and with practically no relationships with children. My mother did not breastfeed me because, at that time, powdered milk was supposed to be the best option for mothers, so breastfeeding for me was not an extension of my parenting philosophy. Of course, I have a lot of friends with kids, but somehow, when I asked for their opinions about how to be a mother, breastfeeding sounded so easy to me that I decided not to read anything or contact any lactation specialists during my pregnancy. Moreover, I decided to pass my two remaining final exams at the university when my baby was born. It seemed so easy. I thought that all babies were like those shown in Johnson & Johnson commercials.

I still remember my third day in the hospital after my beautiful baby was born. Everything was going perfectly well. My husband and

I were happy and exhausted, but I knew that things were going to be all right when we arrived home, or at least that is what we thought.

Alma started crying desperately on that third day. Nobody at the hospital—not her father, not me, not anyone—could comfort her: nothing could except for my breasts. This was, at that moment, just a detail. Then, when time passed, it turned out to be the most interesting tip in the world.

As I said, Alma simply cried and cried all the time. I could never use a seat or trolley because she would quickly burst into tears. Of course, this situation made me think that I was not a good mom to her. If I was, she would have been happy and smiling like the rest of the babies. My first thought was, *"Maybe she would be happier and more relaxed with another mom. Maybe I have to leave this world, and thus someone better than me could give her what she needs."* This was more than baby blues and postpartum depression; I was sure that I was doing things in an incorrect way.

With this entire situation going on, I began to feel that my breasts did not produce enough milk for my little baby. I started working when Alma was 3 months old, and at that moment, I felt that my breasts were dry. Of course, I checked on similar cases on the Internet and surfed on the Web until I found a very interesting site, which led me to La Leche League. There I found the telephone number and email address of one of the Leaders who was supposed to help me.

I still remember that Leader, Ana Clara. I remember how much she talked to me and how much I cried. Ana Clara opened a completely new world to me because she showed to me the very key to my baby and me. I discovered that my milk, my tits, were the connection between my daughter and me. I found out that working at the office was no problem at all because every time I went to the bathroom to extract milk with my hands or with the pump, it made me feel that we were together, embraced by an invisible tie.

So, I changed my mind and stopped trying to avoid, deny, and refuse what I was feeling. I saw myself and Alma in a mirror and discovered that our scars could be healed with my breasts. I saw my past, I saw my pains, and I saw my fears. Our souls were connected. Her name, which means *"soul"* in Spanish, turned out to be my very own soul.

Until that moment, I had been reading and talking to everyone that I knew, but I realized that there was no better book, site, forum, or magazine to read than my little daughter. There was no better psychologist than her. Of course, you have to face your own demons to get rid of them, but what wouldn't you do for your baby?

The most astonishing thing that I learned after having read so much, after having tried every herbal tea, every galactagogue, every domperidone, every metoclopramide, every crazy idea to fill my breasts with milk was that the easiest way was letting my baby suck as much as possible! I still wonder why I looked for the most difficult way. I think that even if breastfeeding is natural, it is not automatic, and moms need, on certain occasions, to listen to their instincts. Of course, your mom, your mother-in-law, your midwife, and your best friend can help, but listening to your deep mammalian instincts is the best way.

I really do not know why modern societies try to change what works perfectly well for our race. If only those food giants would stop interfering with women's lactation. If only those hypocritical attitudes that ban lactating, stretch-marked breasts but encourage sexy and erotic ones would stop. If only we, as women, were not influenced by commercials, by suggestions, by pediatricians. I am sure that societies must evolve, but denying our animal instincts will lead us only to frustration, confusion, and sadness.

Yes, I still breastfeed my 46-month-old Alma. I deeply feel that it is the only way to connect our spirits. By letting her feel that I am always going to be there when she needs me, that there is no clock, no timetable, and no structure for us and for her food, I am bringing up a happy, intelligent, independent, and social girl. We arrived at this point thanks to a lot of people and facts that made us discover that breastfeeding was the best way. In our case, there have been no magical or unique reasons for continuing to breastfeed. We just have.

However, when I see my little girl breastfeeding her doll, rocking her in her arms without any bottle or dummy but instead with her breasts, I can smile and feel that I was able to tell her the secret of motherhood.

I do not want to finish without thanking my husband. He is the best father in the world. Without his support, love, and respect, I would have never been able to breastfeed our daughter for this long. During this period, I made him do so many crazy things to help me breastfeed that I am sure one day we will laugh at them all.

Friend and Foe

Brandy J. Hansen, IBCLC, Normal, Illinois

M y husband had always been pretty supportive of breastfeeding, although not necessarily in a way that shouted to the world about how special or awesome it was. I always knew that he had my back if people talked smack about my nursing the girls or breastfeeding in general. He was just that type of guy. His approach was always more practical than dramatic, and his support was more subtle and manifested in ways, such as letting me sleep in and nurse the baby on the weekends or snuggling and interacting with the girls while they nursed in the early hours of the morning.

As supportive as he was, there hit a point with breastfeeding where he became very vocal about wanting our younger daughter Ripley to stop nursing. I guess that it hit around the middle of her second year and got worse as she approached 2 years. I noticed that he was starting to slip in comments about weaning, and by the time she turned 2, he was getting more aggressive about telling me that he wanted us to start *"taking her off the boob."* I couldn't help being upset at the mention of actively weaning her—Ripley and I were very close, and as I mentioned in my earlier story, I had a really rough pregnancy. I think that was part of why she and I clung to each other and to breastfeeding so much, if that makes sense—something about needing to take time and solidify our trust and comfort in each other.

Knowing that continuing to breastfeed wouldn't cause any harm to her or me made my resolve stronger, and it probably made my anger greater each time my husband mentioned it. My general feeling was that we should let the kids wean themselves when they felt ready. I felt very strongly about not pushing Ripley into it. She was already down to maybe a few times per day by age 2, and I tried to limit nursing visibly in public, so that I could keep my husband comfortable, but she wasn't showing any signs of wanting to go beyond that.

I could see why my husband might be uncomfortable with it, but I thought, *"If he could just put his feelings aside and think about what she wants, he'd feel differently."* I just wasn't willing to force her hand when it came to nursing. After a few attempts at talking about it that mostly ended in me trying to defend my feelings, then crying, and clamming up on the issue, I begged him to stop asking me until after she hit 2, and then we would really start talking about weaning.

Once she went past 2, we did talk about it, and I explained how I kind of viewed his pushing as an affront to my parenting because breastfeeding was what I did—not the only thing, granted—but one thing that I felt that I did really and extraordinarily well. He seemed to understand, but then he got more passive–aggressive in his attempts to get us to stop nursing.

At first, he made little jokes about her being too big to nurse, but then his *"jokes"* began to get more and more hurtful as time wore on—snide, cutting things that really made me upset. The straw that broke the camel's back, so to speak, was when she was about 2 and-a-half. His irritation with nursing had always been directed at me, and I could handle that. Boy, did he use every trick in the book to try and convince me that she needed to stop! He tried blaming her typical 2-year-old crankiness on nursing and said that it was causing behavioral problems (which brought back memories that I'd forgotten of similar comments he'd made once our older daughter Max had nursed for a little over a year). He claimed that I was just doing it because my job as a lactation consultant was about breastfeeding, and I felt like I had to make an example out of her. He even said once, shortly before the incident described here, that he wasn't getting to bond with her because we were nursing so much. I reminded him that nursing never came between him and Max and that breastfeeding wasn't keeping him from Ripley either. This incident, though, was much different than anything I'd seen out of him before.

At this time, Ripley had already been weaning herself slowly—she would go for a couple of days without nursing, then nurse once or twice a day, then stop for another day or two, and so on. While we were putting the kids to bed one night, Max sat in her bed, I was sitting with Ripley on my lap, and we were listening to my husband read the nightly story. Ripley looked at me with this funny little look and politely said, *"Mommy, may I please have 'bub'?"* Of course, I let my shirt open a bit, and she nursed.

My husband then gave us one of the nastiest looks I have ever seen, scoffed loudly, and said, *"It's like you're doing that on purpose—you're nursing her intentionally just to piss me off!"* She kept nursing but gave me kind of a sideways glance.

Astonished, hurt, and incredulous, I looked at him—my lover, my rock, and now my biggest barrier—and hissed lowly, *"I can't believe you just said that in front of her. Do you have any idea what an asshole you're being?!"* After the kids were put to bed, we had words downstairs—accusations about my using nursing to keep Ripley to myself, me being selfish because I wanted to keep nursing, and me using her for my own gain—and that was the last conversation we had for about three days.

On the third night after the bedroom incident, I was getting very close to giving in to his pressure to wean. I was seriously wondering if it was worth this much trouble; if weaning was putting this much pressure between us, what did that say about my priorities in our marriage? Were my kids' rights more important than my husband's wishes and feelings? Was this one of those infamous *"pick your battles"* incidents my mother warned me about, and if so, was it one I should stick with or raise the white flag and surrender in the name of household peace?

When I sat in the rocking chair that evening, I had Ripley on my lap. I was thinking about all this tension, and she asked very politely to bub. Caving a bit, I said, *"You know, baby, one of these days, you're going to be too big to bub."*

"I know," she said.

A bit surprised, I asked, *"How do you know?"*

"Daddy said I too big to bub," she said.

I paused, then asked gently, *"How does that make you feel?"*

"It hurt my heart," she said, pointing to her heart.

I pulled up my shirt, let her latch, and nearly cried. It was at that moment that I got my answer about the battle; it turns out that it wasn't my flag to wave. Later, I went downstairs to the kitchen where my husband was. We still weren't talking. I stood, both hands planted on the counter, and seriously considered whether I should tell him what she had said, whether it really would matter to him, and whether I should just let it be my own secret. I decided to let him have it with both barrels; I told him about our conversation, word for word, and he fell silent. *"Stupid baby—breakin' my heart!"* he said, sniffling a bit.

I didn't hear another word about weaning from him until she was nearly done and that was just as I reported: few and far between nips and nuzzles. Close to her third birthday, she started back with the on-again, off-again feeds until she went for three weeks without latching back on. On November 14, 2011, she sat on my lap and asked one last time, *"Momma, can I bub please?"* and latched on. She suckled a little for a minute but came away only with a mouth full of saliva and a hearty laugh.

I have a lot of training and knowledge about breastfeeding because of my job and lots of experience in encouraging moms to stand their ground when they feel someone is being unsupportive. The night of the heated row with my husband, I needed every bit of that advice and knowledge to defend what I felt I shouldn't have had to defend: the right for my daughter and I to have a close, physical relationship that ended when she was ready.

Ultimately, I knew in my heart that if I caved in to his pressure, I would always regret it. I'm glad that I didn't because, if I had, I would never have realized that as a mom, it will always be my duty to be my children's voice until they can find their own. When they do, they are going to move mountains.

From Child Nurser to Professional Dancer
Pushpa Panadam, Asuncion, Paraguay[5]

In February 2013, my 17-year-old son Jiva José received an offer to join the Ballet Company of Teatro Colon, a prestigious ballet company in Buenos Aires, Argentina. All of a sudden, my husband and I felt that our time of togetherness with our son was drawing to a close. As a family, we were excited for him. It was a wonderful opportunity, and we fully supported and encouraged him. It was a dream come true for him to dance professionally; yet as happy as I was, I was worried: Was he ready to leave home, to be independent at this young age?

I started reflecting on our moments together, his intense need for me, those times when he breastfed. Were these reflections of my coping mechanism? Perhaps. I was thankful that I could revisit those moments as he prepared to leave for another country. Jiva, my second child, was breastfed for more than three years. In fact, I cannot really remember when he actually stopped breastfeeding. However, I could now draw joy and comfort from those precious moments that were made possible by the support that I found in varying forms from my family and friends.

Gayatri, Jiva's older sister, was born in Malaysia, my country. We moved to my husband's home in Paraguay when Gayatri was almost 6 months old. I breastfed her for exactly one year and two months. Yes, I remember clearly because I weaned her suddenly when I learned that I was pregnant again. I felt nausea each time she nursed, and

5   Pushpa thanks Manuel Velázquez, Lisa Gayatri, and Jiva Jose, without whom this story would not have been possible.

at that time, I did not realize that one could continue to breastfeed through pregnancy. Looking back, I can still hear her heart-wrenching cries to nurse, especially to sleep. Instead, she was rocked to sleep by my mother-in-law.

It was different with Jiva. Different in the sense that I felt supported to continue breastfeeding beyond his first year. Jiva was born in 1995 in Asuncion, Paraguay, and I breastfed him exclusively as I did his sister without any problems. I was very clear about exclusively breastfeeding my children and continued to breastfeed when food was introduced in their first year, but the right support at crucial moments made a great difference in my breastfeeding Jiva beyond 2 years and then beyond 3 years.

That needed support came unexpectedly. My husband Manuel, my partner and main support person, learned in the newspaper about La Leche League (LLL)'s Latin American Regional Workshop in Asuncion, Paraguay. That was in August 1996. Manuel asked that I call as he realized that I needed a group that supported breastfeeding. In fact, he told me, *"Call. There is a group which thinks like you!"*

Through that call, I was introduced to a wonderful group of mothers who were sensitive to the needs of their babies and children. I was not very fluent in Spanish at that time, so it was good that I was connected to a Leader who spoke English.

She invited me to their workshop. At the workshop, the Leader Pili Peña nursed her 1-year-old son, who was similar in age to Jiva, as we conversed. She invited me to their monthly support group meetings. It was at that first meeting that I found women nursing their toddlers openly as if it were the most natural thing in the world. Of course, it was and still is.

Seeing these mothers nursing their babies and toddlers gave me the confidence to nurse my 1-year-old openly too. This was important, as my mum-in-law ran a convenience shop from her home, and I often got unwarranted comments regarding breastfeeding my son in her shop. Clients who saw us breastfeeding would say, *"What? Still nursing? He is so big."*

Imagine a 1-year-old being too big to nurse! Perhaps because of those comments, my mum-in-law started to ask when I was going to wean him. I would just say soon. What I learned much later, to my surprise, was that my mother-in-law had breastfed her two sons for more than two years.

The *"soon"* would be after our trip to Malaysia to visit my family at the end of that year. Breastfeeding Jiva, who was then 1½ years old, on the long trip (about 40 hours with four transfers) was easy for us, with no worries about what he should eat or drink.

During a flight, we found ourselves next to a couple with a son about Jiva's age. That baby cried often during the flight while his mother tried desperately to prepare formula with the help of the flight attendants. Her husband, who was trying to calm their son in the meanwhile, was perplexed as to why our son was so calm throughout the journey. My husband, in answer to his query as to why our son did not cry, said, *"His milk is ever ready,"* and explained that Jiva was breastfed. It was easy to calm Jiva during the many flight take-offs by putting him to the breast.

While in Malaysia, we participated in Thaipusam, a yearly Hindu religious festival where devotees fulfill their vows at hilltop temples. In my hometown of Penang, the temple area covers a large open space that caters to the hundreds of people who come to celebrate the festival. My son wanted to nurse because it calmed him, and although I was dressed in a sari, I found a seat, sat, and breastfed him. I was surprised at my mum's reaction to my nursing him there. She, who had been supportive of my breastfeeding (I guess that it was okay but only at home!), became agitated.

"Cover yourself," she told me. *"Can't you wait?"* she asked as I breastfed in the presence of many. Was it because I was exposing my breasts? I remember her standing and looking away from me while I breastfed Jiva, yet the sari top amply covered my breasts.

Reflecting on it now, I realize that if she had understood and accepted that the needs of toddlers came first, it would have helped my mother support me at that time. I say toddler because my mother had traveled to Paraguay when Jiva was born and spent three months caring for me and my daughter while I cared for baby Jiva. I was able to nurse my toddler at the festival that day in Penang, immune to the stares of others, because I had Manuel beside me.

Our breastfeeding experience did not end when we returned to Paraguay after all. In fact, it just made me more determined as I very much enjoyed those moments with my growing child. It was also at that time that I became an LLL Leader Applicant. The training, the friendship, and the LLL library books on breastfeeding and childcare were important resources for me.

As Jiva grew older and understood the comments that people made about him breastfeeding, he would take hold of my hand and say, *"Come, Amma,"* and we would go to our room. He sometimes would ask that I lie down so that he could do his gymnastic nursing, which he loved because he was in total control. Those were fun times. Who would have thought that his agility and flexibility were preparing him for his future dance career?

In 1998, Gayatri, Jiva, and I traveled to Leicester in the United Kingdom to provide support for my youngest sister, who was pregnant with her first child. Once, as we traveled on a bus, he requested to nurse, so I nursed him without any drama. My sister felt uncomfortable, and she asked if I could wait to nurse him until we got back to her house. I just smiled and said, *"No, he needs it now."*

After my niece was born, I helped and supported my sister in breastfeeding her daughter. Jiva would follow me closely if I was near the baby, even at night when I got up to help my sister. He was afraid that the baby wanted his milk!

Later, there was an incident that made me glad that I was still breastfeeding Jiva. This was when he was 4 years old. He was playing on the swing on the patio while I was bringing in the dried clothes. The next thing I knew, I saw him fly off the swing, fall flat onto the concrete floor of the patio, and hit his forehead. I rushed to pick him up, ran to my mother-in-law, and asked what I should do. I was shaking, so afraid and very nervous. My husband was at work. My mother-in-law immediately told me to put him to my breast. I was glad that she asked me to do that; shaking as I was, I just couldn't think what to do. I did what I was told, and he nursed and fell asleep. Then, I called my cousin-in-law, a pediatrician, who told me to keep a close watch on him for the next 24 hours. She said that I would be told to do the same at the hospital.

To my surprise, my husband came home early that evening. He said that he had felt uneasy, and here he found out that something bad had indeed happened. He found Jiva asleep on the sofa and me looking worried. When Jiva woke up, he seemed fine, but we consulted his doctor all the same. It was amazing that my mother-in-law had asked that I nurse him immediately. It was something that I could do at that moment that calmed Jiva and calmed me. What if he had not been a breastfeeding child?

My son continued to breastfeed through kindergarten, although not as often. He would nurse for very short periods and sometimes did not ask for weeks, but mostly when he did, it was at night. Perhaps he was 5 or 6? I cannot really remember when he actually stopped completely asking. Sometimes, it seemed as if he just kissed my nipples. It happened so slowly, and it did not really matter to me.

I remember telling him at times when he asked to nurse that there was no more milk. He would say, *"Of course, there is. If I suck more, the milk will come. You will see."* Just imagine hearing that from a child! He knew that the more he sucked, the more the milk would come.

So, how did Jiva react to the fact that he had breastfed for so long? His teachers knew he had breastfed, and when asked, he would show with his fingers (not speak out) how long he had according to him.

Then, at a live television interview in September 2004, 9-year-old Jiva accompanied his sister, who shared her experience as Paraguay's representative to the Tunza International Children's Conference on the Environment in New London, Connecticut, USA. Gayatri's project was on breastfeeding and the environment. At one point, the interviewer turned to Jiva and asked, *"So, how long did you breastfeed?"* He looked at her straight in the eye and told her, *"Six years."* The interviewer was completely taken aback and asked me as I stood in the sidelines if it was true. What could I do but smile?

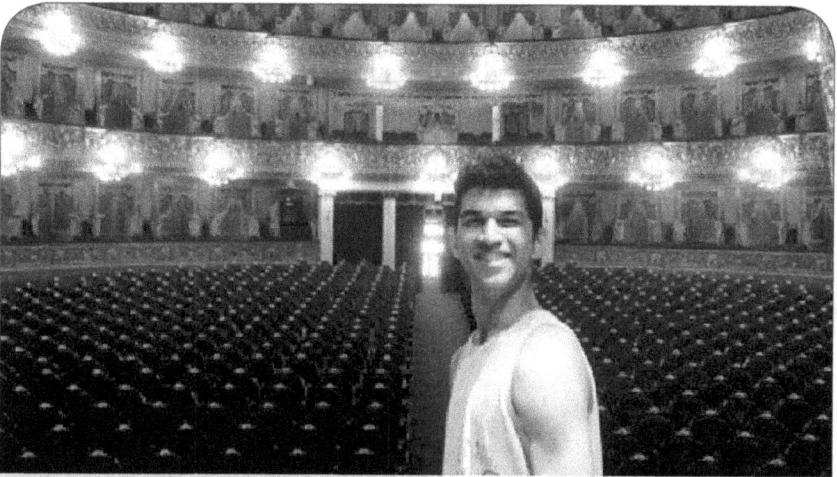

Jiva José Velázquez Panadam in Teatro Colon,
Buenos Aires, Argentina, at the end of his first year.
Photographed by Alejo Joaquín Cano Maldonado, Buenos Aires, Argentina.

It has now been nine months since Jiva began to live on his own. To visit him, it is a bus journey of more than 20 hours. However, we, as his family, are happy and proud of him as he is a disciplined young adult of 18 in a career that he loves: dance. We keep in touch via Skype and Whatsapp almost every day.

Yes, Jiva was ready to leave home at 17. He knows that he is loved, he is secure, and he respects himself and other people. He is able to make decisions, he is gentle and kind, he is capable, he cleans and cooks, and he eats well.

Of course, I should not have worried at all. However, as a mother, I am happy that I have those jeweled moments to hold onto. I am glad that breastfeeding and weaning Jiva as part of a natural process taught me to respect and support him in what he wanted to do as a person when breastfeeding was long over. I could not have done it without the total support and respect that I received from my husband and the others around me.

Nursing for Me

Libby Jewell, Howell, Michigan

My daughter fell asleep while she was nursing last night. Well, at least for a few minutes. It's been at least a couple of years since she's done that...wait a couple of years?! Wow, I guess we have been nursing for a long time!

Lucy will be 4 in December. She has been sick this week with a little cold, probably from preschool, which she started in September. Actually, we've all been sick this week. So, I was snuggling on the couch with my husband and getting ready to fall asleep in front of a movie when, around midnight, I heard some whimpers. My body tensed up, ready to spring, the way it has ever since she was born. Then, after a few minutes of quiet, my body relaxed, and I was hoping against hope that she would just soothe herself and go back to sleep. No luck. When I heard more whimpering, I jumped up, irritated and grumbling to my husband, and went up to check on her. As soon as I saw her, my heart melted the way it always does, even through the irritation.

"How ya doing, buddy?"

"Not good."

"Aww, how come?"

She pointed to her throat.

I melted even more. *"Do you just want to spend the rest of the night in momma's bed?"*

She nodded, slid out of her bed, and took my hand.

"Can I nurse, Momma?"

"Of course, buddy."

Chapter 4

I'm a sucker, a pushover. We slid under the sheets and got cozy, and I knew that we were both in for a terrible night of sleep.

Nursing at night actually drives me really crazy. I can't sleep through it. She sleeps fitfully and wants to nurse all the time, but then she never really goes into a deep sleep while she's nursing. Flashbacks of sleep deprivation, of the girl who didn't sleep through the night for 18 months and nursed every 2 hours, and of sleeping on a mattress in her room together, give me a shiver of déjà vu. Plus, she has to play with (tweak, pinch, roll—ouch!) one nipple while she's nursing the other one. It is totally aggravating. She nurses more when she's feeling vulnerable, sick, sad, or upset. So, this was one of those times.

Once the sucking slowed down and her breathing became even, I finally said, *"Okay, buddy, you need to roll over and go to sleep now."* It was 1 a.m. Reluctantly, she turned over, and eventually, she fell asleep. She woke again at 6:22 a.m. *"Can I nurse, Momma?"*
I sighed.
We dozed fitfully until 8 a.m. when my husband finally came wandering up from the couch. *"How did you guys sleep?"* he asked.
"Ugh," I said.

Last night got me thinking about my own personal journey of breastfeeding. It has not been easy, but it really has not been too hard, either. When I think about the support I have had, I feel very satisfied. My husband Jeff has always been supportive of nursing, even when he perhaps wished the whole thing would just stop. I certainly did not foresee how difficult nursing might be on a marriage.

It is a complete bond, one that demands a high level of attention to my daughter, and one that sometimes takes away from time with my husband.

Once we got past 3, however, the difficulties of nursing seemed to gradually fade. Perhaps it's because we don't nurse as often (we will often go a day or two without nursing at all) or simply because she is more independent.

I would say that I've also gotten a fair amount of support from my family too. We don't necessarily talk about it all the time, but I've never actually had anyone say anything negative about it. The closest I got was when I was at a museum with my in-laws. My daughter was having a tantrum, and I sat down to nurse her on a public bench. I felt on the defensive—after all, I've read lots of stories about women who have endured a disapproving eye for breastfeeding in public. I remember almost wanting someone to say something, like I wanted to have that fight, just so I'd have a good story, but no one did.

So, after a minor rocky start as a newborn, my daughter has been successfully nursing for almost four years. My husband has been extremely supportive, even what I would call sacrificial, to support me in my quest to continue nursing. My family members (even my in-laws!) have been supportive (my sister-in-law even attended a national latch-on in public with me), and my friends have ranged from being totally supportive to really not caring one way or the other. I've had the chance to have rational conversations with those who think that it's slightly strange to nurse someone to this age and even convinced a few of its benefits.

As I pondered all this, I began to wonder, *"So, if everyone in my life has been so wonderful about this, why do I ever feel negative about breastfeeding at all?"*

For me, it comes down to a couple of things: me throwing myself into parenting (sometimes too much) and my daughter being what I would call an intense child. Ever since she was born and was so fussy that she didn't sleep for about 18 hours after I gave birth, she has always demanded a lot out of me as a parent. She is intense, I am intense, and our relationship together is intense.

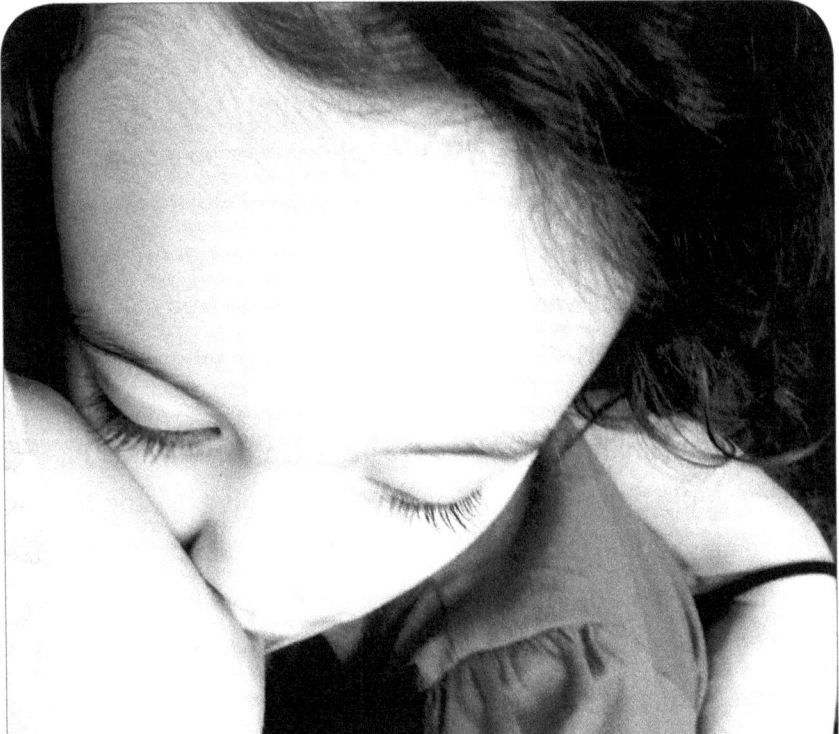

Libby nursing 3-year-old Lucy at the doctor's office after she got a "throat poke" (a swab for strep throat).

In addition, I work almost full-time and in several different roles. I have very little time for myself. I actually went through a period about a year ago where I considered trying to wean her. She was about 2½, and I was finding the whole process really agitating. I even borrowed some sage from a friend, which is apparently supposed to dry up your milk, but I could just never go through with it. I kept putting it off until one day I realized that I was not ready to stop.

I've been mulling this over for the last several days. Right now, it's almost 1 a.m. I had a long week of work on top of a difficult week of parenting and dealing with almost-4-year-old behavior issues, and the answer suddenly became clear: breastfeeding a child is a lot of work! The commitment required to breastfeed this long can be difficult, inconvenient, awkward, burdensome, demanding, and exhausting. I've been doing this for four years, and I am tired!

I almost feel guilty admitting this. I have all this support. I don't have any earth-shattering story about how terrible someone was to me when I tried to breastfeed in public, and I know so many women who couldn't breastfeed their babies or had to stop earlier than they wanted, and here I am, talking negatively about it.

When I was in the throes of early newborn life—when I was going through postpartum blues and was sleep-deprived, overwhelmed, and physically sore—I once had a friend tell me that when her son was a newborn, she got to the point of being so sleep-deprived and feeling overwhelmed with his crying that she felt like throwing him in the garbage can. I know, I know—it's awful. Of course, she would have never done anything of the sort, but it surprised me so much when she said that. It was such a stark relief to hear someone admit that she was not a perfect parent, and how freaking hard having a newborn could be that I burst out laughing. Here was a real mom who was admitting that parenting could suck sometimes, and it was okay to say that out loud.

I say all this about nursing in the same vein. Sometimes, I feel like I'm going to crawl out of my skin while she's nursing. Sometimes, I find it completely annoying and aggravating. Sometimes, I want to yell and scream and say, *"Aahh! Get off of me!"*

However, as I've been writing this, a realization has slowly material-ized for me. I understand that the main reason I am still breastfeeding after four years...drumroll please...is for me. Yes, I do it for her and for us, of course, but I'm proud of the fact that I'm still nursing. I'm proud of the nourishment and protection that it offers her. I enjoy the bonding, the closeness, the sweetness, and the connection, even through the aggravation, annoyance, and difficulty.

I recently read an article about a woman in her early 50s who was still breastfeeding her kindergartener. Before I had my daughter, I might have thought that was a little weird, but now I think it's the coolest thing in the world. Today, I know in my heart that I will let her nurse for as long as she wants—for her, for us, and for me.

Disregarding Disapproval
Helen, Redditch, Worcestershire, United Kingdom

My son, whom I continue to breastfeed, started school today. He is 4½ years old. I don't know how many children are still breastfed when they start school in the United Kingdom, but I guarantee that he'll be the only one in his class of 30. Like many others, I am feeding him in secret now—in secret from my close family, from most of my friends (except the most enlightened of my *"boobie"* friends), from health professionals, including my general practitioner, who recently prescribed me strong pain killers not knowing I was too embarrassed to say that I was breastfeeding a 4-year-old. I never filled the prescription because I knew that I couldn't take them. The last health professional I shared this information with was my health visitor when my son was almost 3, and her response was simply to ask me, *"When are you going to stop?"*

The last time I fed in public, he had just turned 4, and it was at our local breastfeeding support group at a children's center. He had bumped his head and was upset, and pulling at my top, he asked for *"milky."* I wanted to calm him quickly, and I knew this would be the quickest way. I thought that if I couldn't feed him at a breastfeeding support group, where could I? I did feel really uncomfortable though.

I know that we are already beyond the worldwide average age for breastfeeding cessation, let alone the United Kingdom's, whose average must be more easily measured in months rather than years! I continue to feed because my son still asks for it. I am happy to let him for lots of reasons (see Editor's Note on page #269.)

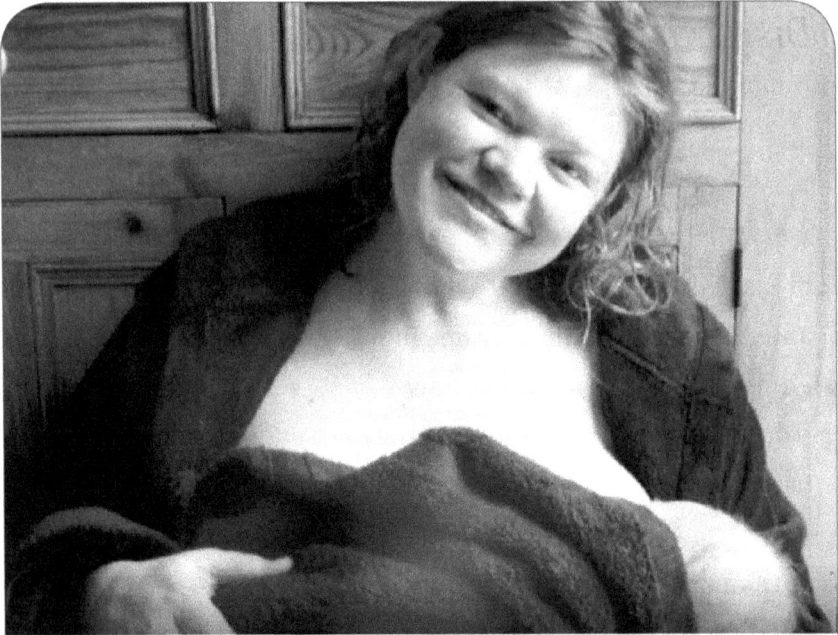

Helen and her son during his first feeding at the breast after a home water birth.

I was discussing breastfeeding duration with a breastfeeding mother recently. I asked her if she had any idea what the average worldwide age for weaning was. She replied, *"Four months."* She was shocked (and almost looked appalled) when I said it was 4 years. I was shocked by her reaction too. It made me realize how out of the ordinary our breastfeeding relationship was and how many people might not find it acceptable anymore (see Editor's Note on page #269.)

I remember that I used to share those prejudices, too. I remember feeding my eldest son at 4 months on a flight to Australia. I sat next to a woman who was also breastfeeding her 22-month-old. At the time, I thought her child was too old to be breastfed. I did not say it, of course, but I wonder if my face shared my thoughts nonetheless. I wish that I could go back and talk to that mother and tell her what an amazing thing she was doing for her daughter by feeding her in public. I'd tell her that I hoped we would still be feeding when my son was her daughter's age.

Facebook is a safe place for people to openly share their prejudices behind an anonymous avatar. I have shared my extended breast-feeding experience there, and the reactions from many people have demonstrated how so many find something sinister in breastfeeding older children. If you've ever breastfed an older child, you know that there's no way you can force a child who does not want to. If only it could be so easily controlled by the mother!

There have been times when I've thought, *"I've had enough."* Some mornings, I feel so touched out. I'm not a great morning person anyway, and having a little person all over you early in the morning can be overwhelming sometimes. Then, add to that the constant nipple twiddling with the one he's not feeding from, and it can drive me nuts.

So, this notion that it is the mother who does not wish to let go or, worse, that in some way it is abusive of the mother is utter nonsense. However, our society, including schools and health professionals, has little or no experience of extended feeding like ours, and some even frown on it and consider it to be damaging for the child. Of course, if we all continue to do it in secret, attitudes will never change.

My son still asks for milky. I have been practicing *"don't offer, don't refuse"* since he was 3, and he still asks. Not every night or every morning, but more often than not, he does ask. Sometimes, he asks in the day when we are together if he is upset or tired. He has gone through phases of asking less and less, and at times, I think that he is going to stop.

We have had extended periods apart, up to five days once, but every time, he comes back to it. Then, at other times, the requests increase again. The most interesting part is how my milk supply just keeps adjusting to whatever his pattern is at the time—clever boobies!

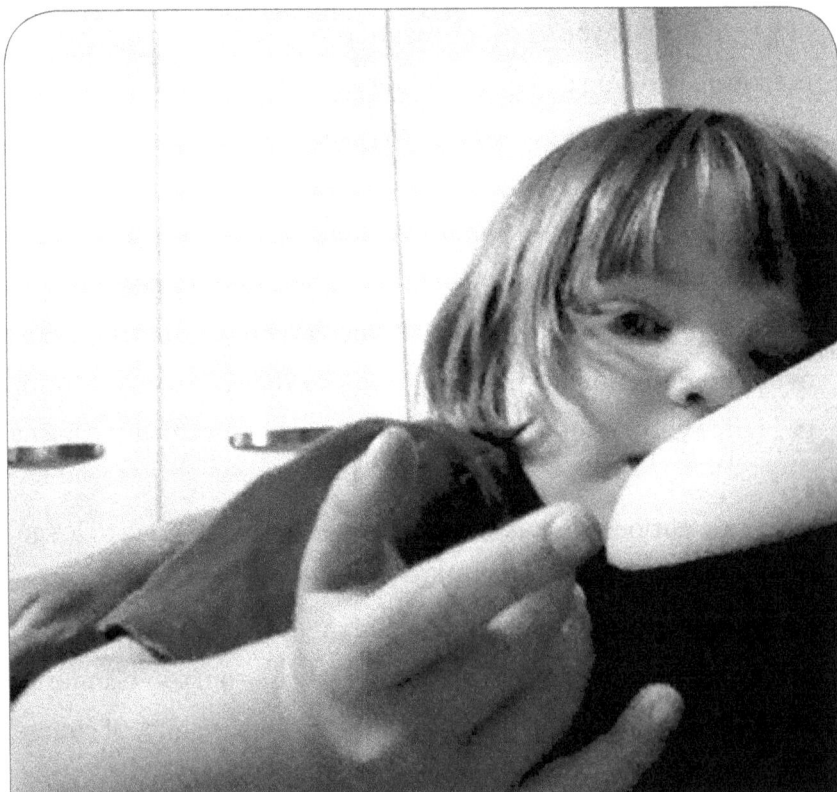

Helen's son breastfeeding at age 4 while shooting a "Spidey" web.

My son has never needed antibiotics, has never been hospitalized, and has only been to the doctor once or twice maybe. I can barely remember taking him or even what it was for. He's never had a day sick from nursery or school. His extraordinary health record is one of the main reasons that I continue to breastfeed him.

My eldest son stopped at 11 months. On reflection, it was a nursing strike, but I didn't know then what I do now. Two weeks later, we were in the hospital with his first asthma attack. He's been hospitalized three more times since then, and he suffers from chronic eczema.

I can't go back and change what I did then, however guilty I feel. He had formula at 3 months, and I stopped breastfeeding altogether before 12 months. I believe that this most likely contributed to his allergies, eczema, and asthma. We have a family history of all these things, and I wish that I had been better informed then about the risks of formula and the benefits of breastfeeding beyond the first year because of our family history.

I want to give my youngest the very best chance of a healthy future, and breastfeeding has a dose-related protective factor. Given the fact that I have fed this long, I have resigned myself to the fact that he will most likely self-wean. I am comfortable with that. I might try and gently encourage him when he turns 5, but I will not force him if he's not ready. Unless, of course, I change my mind and no longer wish to do it myself. It's a mother's prerogative! I don't believe that there's anything wrong with a mother choosing to stop for herself. In nature, many mothers wean by force. I do believe breastfeeding works best when both parties are happy with it.

My son is obviously not ashamed or embarrassed as he does ask for milky by name in front of people. He also puts his hands down my top for comfort quite often in public. I just gently pull his hand out and ask him not to do that. I don't make a big fuss about it or draw particular attention to it. I know children who still do this even though they stopped breastfeeding years before. For my son, it is a form of comfort, although sometimes pulling my top down to reveal my bra is not always appropriate, so I ask him not to do it. I will give him a cuddle instead, and he is usually placated with that.

I love breastfeeding my son, but not everyone around me loves it quite so much. My husband doesn't seem very happy about it. I don't understand why feeding our son offends him so much. He tries to use not feeding him as a punishment for his more challenging behaviors. *"You don't deserve that,"* he'll say, as if it is a reward.

To my son, it's not a reward for anything. It's just milky. I don't want our son thinking that he is doing something wrong or that it is being used as a form of discipline either. To hear his daddy say, *"You're too old for that now"* or *"What are you letting him do that for?"* is hurtful. When such prejudice comes from within your own immediate family, it's really upsetting.

I know women with younger babies hear comments such as *"Are you still doing that?"* or *"Isn't it time you stopped that?"* from family members. I appreciate that we are at the more extreme end for breastfeeding, but it feels just as hurtful to hear those words now as if I'd heard them at 6 weeks or 6 months. I know that my son will not feed forever and may even stop very suddenly.

Breastfeeding takes such a great deal of effort, commitment, and determination to get started in the beginning and to keep going.

Everyone expects you to breastfeed a newborn baby and to commit everything to it. So, why, at some later arbitrary age, is everyone so obsessed with when you are going to stop? Perhaps this is why I pretend that I already have!

One for the Books
Suzanne P. Reese, Ramona, California

Like most mothers I know, I wanted to breastfeed. Other than the basic putting-the-baby-to-the-breast advice, I didn't know much about how it was going to happen. I had very few preconceived ideas about nursing. Would I do it in public? I didn't know. How long would we nurse? I wasn't certain, but a year was my initial goal.

We had a bit of a rough start. I had milk imbalance, and that caused extreme gastro-intestinal distress for my girl.[6] She screamed for the first 17 weeks of her life. I was sure that it was causing brain damage to her—and to all of us. It took me talking to the right lactation consultant to find out what was wrong and what we could do to remedy it. I miss those first few weeks and have often wished that I could go back with the knowledge that I have now. I feel like I missed out on that newborn bliss that a lot of moms talk about. Heck, I spent much of my life studying that newborn bliss, and I missed out. It felt so unfair. However, what I could not have known was where we'd be today, and what I realize now is that I am fortunate beyond words.

I was a superproducer, and so once my milk was balanced out, I was able to nurse my girl and provide milk for another brother and sister who were having trouble with formula. That was blessing number one. The next blessing is a great fortune that keeps on giving.

Over the years, we've had our share of minor breastfeeding challenges, like a couple of bouts of mild mastitis, milk blisters, raw

---

6   Please see http://www.llli.org/faq/foremilk.html for a full explanation of foremilk/hindmilk imbalance and how it can affect breastfeeding and the baby.

nipples when her teeth came in, and phases of what felt like nonstop nursing, which can be exhausting, but here we are still going strong for her age.

Last year, when she was just turning 4, I was going through some dental issues. My dentist recommended that I have an amalgam filling replaced. There was some significant cracking, and I was in a lot of pain. It was time to address the issue. The dentist was quite set on me weaning my girl. I thought that a clinician telling me that it was time to wean her would be welcome news. She was nearly 4, we'd had an excellent run, and it was time, wasn't it?

When I arrived home from that appointment, I was a mess. I realized that since our girl was our one and only child and since we had decided that we'd let her wean in her own time, the fact that somebody, even a clinician, was dictating when she'd wean was devastating. I was beside myself in grief over the notion that I'd have to tell her she couldn't nurse any longer. I thought of all of the benefits of nursing that she would lose, and then, I thought of what we would lose together, and I simply couldn't do it. I had to find another way.

I found a holistic practitioner, who helped me prepare for the procedure. Even though this dentist was trained and certified in the safe removal of amalgam fillings, I knew that I needed help to reduce what little exposure I was going to have to the mercury that was going to escape. I had the filling replaced and the tooth repaired, and our nursing was never interrupted. I never even mentioned it to my dentist. Balance had been restored.

We are approaching a year from that procedure, and my girl is now about to turn 5. Yes, 5! Last year, before that dental procedure, I asked her if she was interested in stopping nursing. Even after explaining to her why, she let me know that it simply was not an option. This year, I'm delighted to not have a reason to have that discussion with her, and our little family is just fine with where we are.

Fortunately, no one has ever challenged our nursing practices, either privately or publicly, and I have rarely ever used a cover and never felt the need to hide out in a bathroom. I have a tribe of mama friends who are like-minded, and some of us are still going strong as our children approach 4 and 5 years. Other family and mama friends of mine simply accept it, and while I don't go around announcing it, I don't hide it either.

Our girl is one of the healthiest and most well-adjusted little people we know. She's a delight to be around. She is social, makes friends easily, and enjoys people, and she is deeply compassionate. There are no signs, outward or otherwise, that indicate that a full-term nursing relationship with me is not benefitting her. As for us, her parents, it's simply not about us. It's about her. We are not bothered by it. At this point, she only nurses at night and in the morning, at dozing off and at waking up. Sure, there are nights and mornings when she nurses more, and then, there are nights and mornings when she doesn't nurse at all because she's just that exhausted from a busy day or because we are up early and ready to get the day going, so there just isn't time. Either way, it's fine. This will not last forever. That's right, just like many other things, this will not last forever. This summer, she asked to sleep in her own bed in her own room.

There was no previous talk about it. It was just something that she had decided one day. When I asked her why, she said *"Because I'm a big girl now."* For that reason, we are content with her navigating this train because I imagine that one day she will decide she's too big of a girl to nurse anymore.

It's a journey I never expected to still be on, and I'm happy I'm here with her. I feel deeply fortunate and blessed to be able to share such safety, trust, love, and intimacy with my child. I feel honored that it's a relationship that she still wants with me. I cherish every moment but am mindful that this is about her. I rarely offer her milk. Rather, I wait for her to ask for it. Sometimes, we don't say anything at all, and it just happens. At this point, she nurses at night during bedtime stories until she falls asleep and in the morning upon waking. If there is a routine about it, that's it.

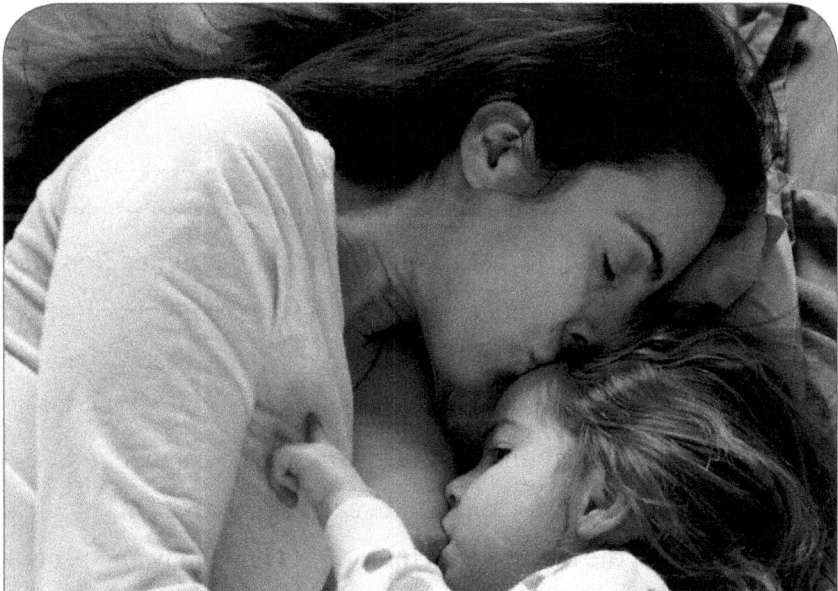

Suzanne and Anika. Photo by Doug Reese.

When she was an infant, I knew that I wanted to nurse her for a year. Upon approaching a year, I decided that since things were going so well, two years was my next goal. At that time, people started asking me how long I planned to nurse, and I'd say *"Well, two years is my goal, but I don't see any signs of her slowing down, so I don't know, we'll see."* By the time she turned 3, people stopped asking, and we weren't nursing in public much anymore, so it was rarely a topic of conversation. When she turned 4, I think that most people assumed we'd stopped, and the people who knew either supported it fully or just respected where we were with it.

Certainly, there are people I don't bring it up with. It's simply not worth it, and it would serve no purpose. Now that we are looking at five years and there is still no sign of her losing interest, I really don't know how long this will last, but it will be up to her. My husband supports whatever is good for her, and together, we support what is clearly working.

I love knowing that no matter what, I can still provide for her a place that represents everything good and balanced in her world. I love knowing that she gets a nutritional and immune boost as a bonus. I love looking at her at such close range, remembering her as an infant, and knowing that I never imagined then that we would be where we are today. I love knowing that this is normal for her. She knows no controversy about full-term nursing. I know that this will not last forever, and so I appreciate each moment of this now-rare relationship in the history of mankind, and I'm happy and proud to know that this is one for the books—even literally so!

Chapter 5

Challenging Situations and Special Needs

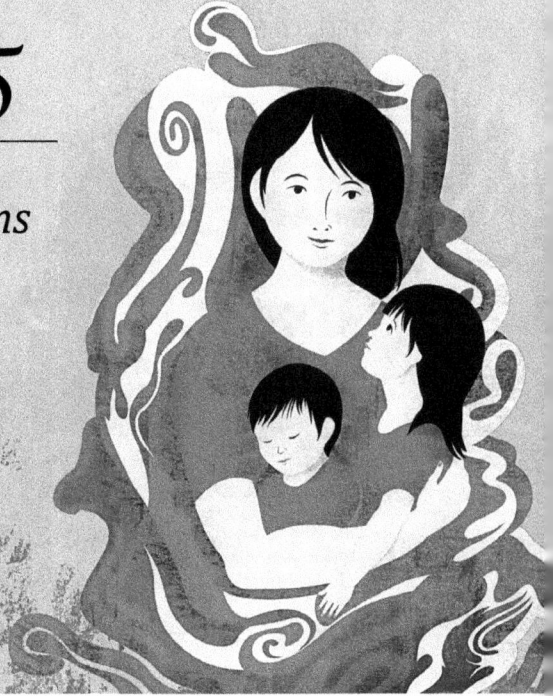

We often hear miracle stories of breastfeeding, about how breast milk is a wonderful, cure-all substance. However, the world is not a perfect place. Breastfed kids still get sick and injured. They are neurotypical and autistic. They are amazingly healthy or they get allergies, eczema, and other typical maladies. Their mothers still deal with stress, both physical and emotional. In other words, they are all human. In these situations, continuing to breastfeed can be a challenge, but it can also be a balm to soothe an otherwise overwhelming situation.

Yes, She's 4, and Yes, She's Still Breastfeeding
Diana Cassar-Uhl, Cornwall, New York[7]

This is Gabriella. She's my youngest daughter, and she turned 4 in December.

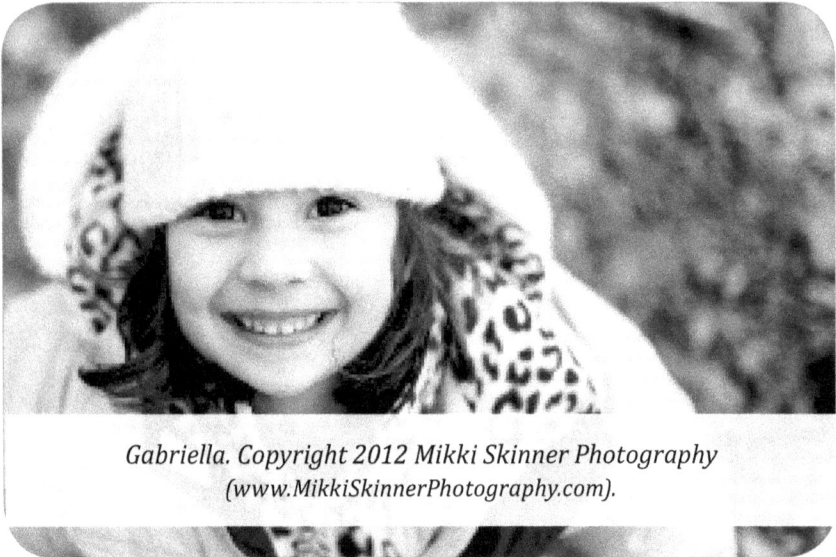

*Gabriella. Copyright 2012 Mikki Skinner Photography
(www.MikkiSkinnerPhotography.com).*

Two weeks after her fourth birthday, Gabriella underwent a 3-hour craniofacial surgery to resolve a rare birth defect. Two pediatric neurosurgeons and a pediatric plastic surgeon cut open my little girl's head in an incision that wrapped from ear to ear. They pulled her scalp and most of her face down and scraped dermoid tissue from the bone between her beautiful eyes, reaching into the suture line to ensure my baby does not have to deal with the invasion of foreign tissue into her brain later in her life.

---

[7]   This story is reprinted from a post on May 11, 2012 on Diana's blog, *normal, like breathing,* which can be found at http://dianaibclc.com/2012/05/11/yes-shes-4-and-yes-shes-still-breastfeeding/. It was also printed in the journal *Clinical Lactation* (2012, Volume 3, Issue 3, pages 119–122), which can be found at http://www.clinicallactation.org/content/blog-watch-yes-shes-4-and-yes-shes-still-breastfeeding.

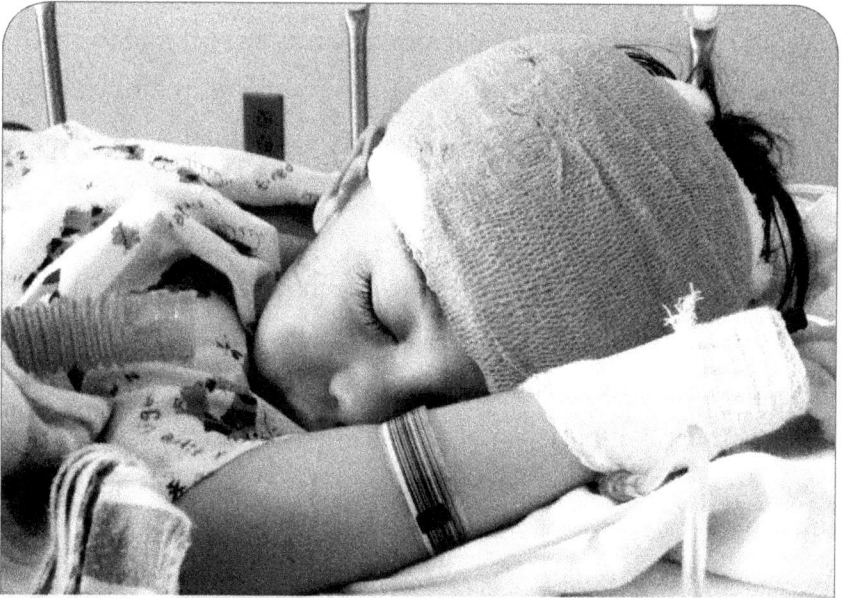

Gabriella, feverish and still sleepy in the recovery room.
©2012 Diana Cassar-Uhl.

It took her a long time to wake up. She ran a little fever in response to the anesthesia and the incredible shock to her system from having her face taken off. Gabriella was so, so brave and compliant, letting the nurses adjust the tubes and probes that were all over her in the recovery room, contented to rest if I held her hand.

We were admitted to her room later in the afternoon, after the recovery nurses felt comfortable letting her go. Gabriella was starting to wake up, and was so happy to see her brother and sister when they came to visit the children's hospital. She was excited to show them the big fire truck to play on and the rooms filled with toys and activities. With five days until Christmas, Santa Claus found some time to bring presents to the children in the hospital, and Gabriella was delighted.

But the morphine made her sick. She was hungry and thirsty, but even ice chips made her throw up. *"I don't want to throw up again, Mamma,"* she told me in her tiny, weak voice. *"I think nursies will help me. Can I nurse?"*

I had anticipated this moment in the months leading up to Gabriella's surgery. Her siblings had each weaned before their fourth birthdays, and I expected that Gabriella would do the same. I half-hoped I would have breastfeeding as a tool to help my little girl through her most difficult life experience to date, but the rest of me worried that she might not wean, and I would find myself on the defensive.

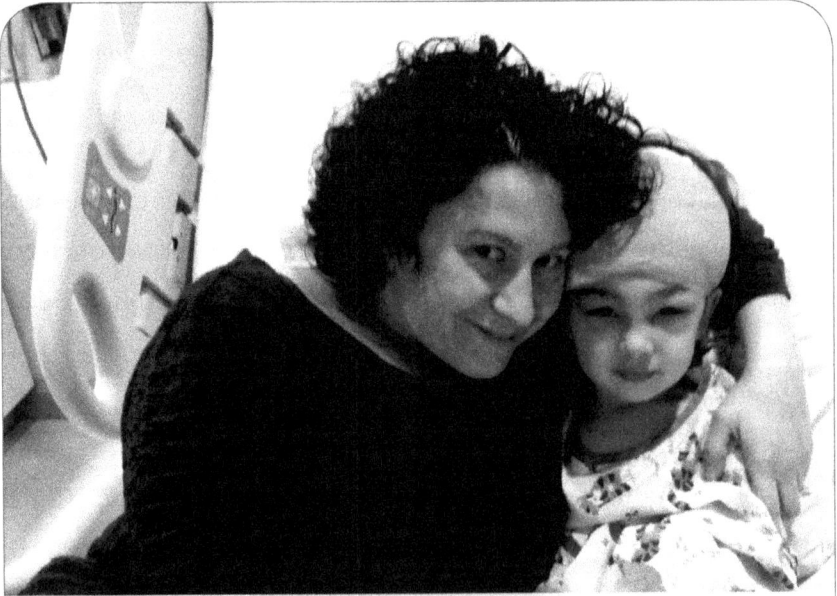

Gabriella and her mamma after napping with nursies.
©2012 Diana Cassar-Uhl.

You see, we live in a time and place where we would rather see a magazine teeming with images of scantily clad women on a beach than a mother breastfeeding her child on a bench. A toddler who climbs into his mother's lap to breastfeed is viewed as stunted and spoiled; his mother is accused of being a slave, or, worse, a pedophile.

I worried that even the healthcare professionals charged with my daughter's healing would strike me down if I comforted her at my breast. I thought about how I might carry Gabriella, in her little hospital gown with happy tigers romping around on it and her IV line, into the not-so-clean, poorly lit bathroom in her room and let her nurse, with the door closed, while I sat on the toilet.

I considered whether I might just nurse her in her bed and receive any confrontations that came our way, praying that none of the staff were so ignorant of normal human biology as to call Child Protective Services in to investigate us. This anxiety came on top of the worry that we hadn't taken care of everything through our insurance, that my job might place unreasonable demands on me when my child needed me the most, that maybe something unexpected would happen during the surgery and my joyful little girl would emerge from it changed...or not emerge at all.

"Yes, darling. Mamma will nurse you."

We arranged her IV line so that neither of us would be on top of it. We laughed when the automatic movement in the mattress, intended to change the position of the patient to prevent bedsores, surprised us as we got settled in to nurse. Her eyes were puffy with fluid that was draining downward from her head, but I could see the relief in them. It didn't matter that we were on a plastic sheet in a noisy hospital ward with narcotic-induced nausea (hers) and utter exhaustion (mine). She latched on, and we were home, safe, and together. Gabriella nursed to sleep, and I drifted off too, for the first time in days.

The shift nurse came in to check Gabriella's vitals when she was still attached to me. She smiled and asked, *"She's holding that down OK, I take it?"* I made a joke about there not being much there anymore, but added *"She doesn't seem to mind."* The nurse didn't challenge me or attack. She didn't accuse me of molesting my sweet girl.

Yesterday, *Time* magazine[8] released its controversial cover photo of a mother and her preschooler. The reaction to that cover was often quite cruel in their descriptions of mother and child.

I am thankful my children, at 9, 7½, and 4, are unaware of what the society around them supposes about their lives. They all remember breastfeeding; they still seek comfort in me, their mother. The foundation is there for an enduring, loving relationship. Being *Old Enough to Ask for It*[9] doesn't forbid a child from receiving comfort from his mother, however that mother chooses to comfort her child. The older child isn't breastfeeding all day or to meet nutritional needs; he's nursing a few times a week because he still needs that *"home base"* connection to his mother, and breastfeeding has provided that basis since the moment he was born. The preschooler who still breastfeeds goes to school with your children, but she doesn't talk about nursing or cry for nursies at rest time; she behaves in

8   From *Time Magazine*, May 21, 2012. See the cover at http://lightbox.time.com/2012/05/10/parenting/#1

9   The blog post *Old Enough to Ask for It* on *normal, like breathing* can be found at http://dianaibclc.com/2011/02/24/old-enough-to-ask-for-it/.

age-appropriate, developmentally normal ways (and if she doesn't, breastfeeding isn't exacerbating whatever the issue is). Breastfeeding my 4-year-old, postoperative child wasn't disgusting, it was normal. Nursing her back to sleep a few nights ago when she woke up in the middle of the night wasn't indulging her, it was loving her the way she has come to expect to feel love and comfort from me, her mother.

Gabriella looks back on her time at *"the hospital hotel"* with smiles. The hair that was shaved to allow the *"boo-boo"* is shorter than the rest of her hair and a little hard to control at five months postop, but she puts on a headband and gets on her way. She experienced no emotional trauma and has no lingering fears or worries about visiting doctors or being subject to tests (she spent nearly 2 hours awake in the noisy tube for a full spinal MRI just a few months ago, in fact). Might Gabriella be so confident and stable, even in the face of tremendous adversity, if she wasn't still breastfeeding? Perhaps she would be...but I'm thankful she and I know what's best for her today, and I'm committed to ensuring that families are not deprived of accurate information about the normality of breastfeeding an older child.

Happy and Healthy with Chronic Low Milk Supply

Ivy, Central Florida

I have chronic low milk supply and a need to power-pump for two days to provide each of my two children with just 2 ounces of my precious milk. I wish that I could say what chronic low milk supply is exactly and why or how it came about for me. Mostly, I cannot do any of those things because neither I nor my children have any of the markers that would explain why I don't lactate more.

In the past, I've worked with Denise Punger, an amazing doctor on the east coast of Florida, to discuss symptoms and reasons. I had an ultrasound of my breast tissue in an attempt to locate possible physical reasons for this condition, and have researched and consumed nearly every herb and galactogogue that I could in an attempt to bring about a normal supply.

Ultimately, it is my hope that both our struggles and successes can help others have an easier time navigating low-milk-supply issues. It sure seems to have brought about an extraspecial connection between myself and my extended nursling.

Because of this chronic low supply, I used a supplemental nursing system (SNS) to provide formula and eventually cow's milk at the breast to my second son from the time he was 7 days old until he was 35 months old. Around the time he was about 18 months old, I heard a story of a local mom who nursed her son at 3½ years old. At that time, my older son was almost 3, and I had similar low-milk-supply issues with him, with the biggest difference being that he refused to nurse with the supplementer, and I sadly stopped power pumping for mere milliliters when he around 11 weeks old.

When I saw this story, I was having a hard time imagining how nursing a super-busy toddler could work out, let alone how I could do it while maintaining our special circumstances and SNS use. I already felt pretty great about actually making it past the six-month mark since I wasn't sure that we'd even make it to a couple of weeks, let alone 18 months. I brought this up to my husband one night while we were making dinner. I had no thought that he would be adverse to extended nursing. To my surprise, he turned to me and said, *"That's a little old isn't it? You'll only be nursing our son until he's 2 years old anyway."*

Now, my husband isn't often firm or pushy in demeanor, and this caught me off guard, especially since he was privy to all of the frustration and hard work we had to do to even be nursing this time around. Feelings of anger and rage welled up in me in response to his offhanded comment, but I took a deep breath and looked at my sweet nursling across the room, and a sudden peace came over me. I turned and calmly said, *"I haven't asked him when he plans on weaning, and he's not talking much anyway, so good luck with a response on that one. I figure he'll let me know, and we'll work together on that, just the way we've worked so hard to make using the SNS successful. This is a relationship that I started, and I won't be the one walking away without agreement."* I think my husband caught on quickly to my unhappiness, even through my calm words, and decided to forgo any further discussion on it. Even though I was able to keep quite calm about it, that conversation was stressful for me, and for quite some time, I had visions of feeling pressured to stop nursing.

About a year later, it came up again. We used to travel off and on for several months with my husband's work and would live in our travel trailer at RV parks close to his work sites. One cold and late night while we were relocating from Nashville to Chicago, we were far from a suitable location to stay overnight, so we pulled into a Walmart parking lot to do our nightly sleep routine with our boys. As my husband hurried to hook up propane to boil water for warm milk to put into our SNS, I sat holding a 2½-year-old toddler who was ready to nurse to sleep. My mind wandered to our conversation, which had happened a year or so ago, and I asked my husband if he remembered what he had said about weaning at 2. He answered, *"Yes, and I figure as long as he's happy and healthy, that's all that really matters."*

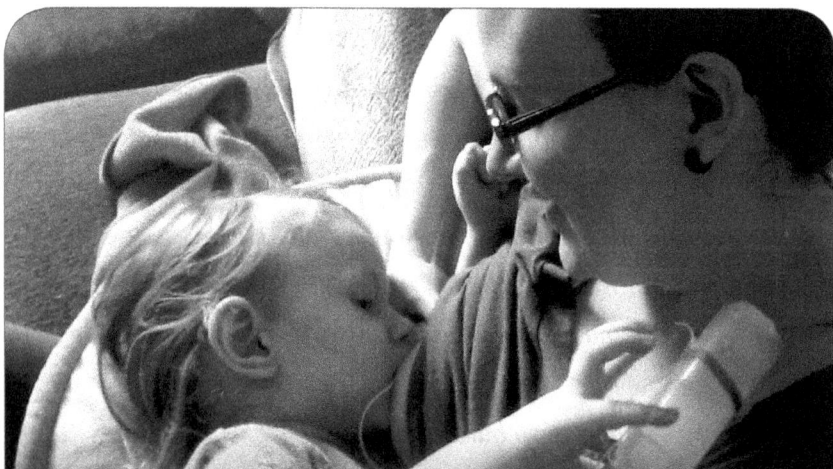

Toddler "gymnurstics" made nursing extra-interesting for Ivy while her little one investigated his SNS.

Just one month before he turned 3, my little guy told me directly that he didn't want to use his *"num num bottle"* at that nursing session. It began with him saying no just for his morning feedings, and then within a week or so, he refused it for every feeding, although we had been using it at waking, naps, and bedtime. I was fearful that this meant that our nursing relationship would be ending soon since most of his intake was from the supplementer. In fact, my little guy has continued to nurse and has been weaning me gently for at least eight months now. Thankfully, I can't even begin to predict when the end will actually come around. I have made sure to let my husband know that it is apparently typical around the world for kids to self-wean after 4 years of age (see Editor's Note on page #269.)

There are often little anniversary moments that cause me to pause and reflect on just how long this nursing journey of ours might last. Every chance we get to nurse is a gift that my son gives to me at this point. Today, my son is a week away being from 3 years 7 months old, and he just interrupted me to nurse as I'm typing this story. These moments are sweet because they happen so few and far between these days. He may ask to use the SNS once or twice a month and probably nurses only three to six times a week, but he still remains in very close contact with his num nums. As hard as it has been to maintain a nursing relationship with a chronically low supply, I know that dealing with differing opinions and working through nursing struggles alongside my husband has definitely brought us closer. He's very accepting of my interactions with other moms who are having issues and just need to chat and hear that they're not alone. It's clear that our nursing experience as a family is allowing us to help others on their path and to heal along the way.

More than Just Milk

Sarah Morris Lin, Santa Clara, California

I never would have imagined that I would be nursing an almost 4-year-old. Not because I don't believe in full-term nursing, but rather because I never thought I would be able to nurse my son in the first place. When my son was 5 weeks old, I found out that I most likely had insufficient glandular tissue (IGT). IGT means that the amount of milk-making tissue in a woman's breasts is too small (to varying degrees) and that she will not make enough milk, no matter how much breast stimulation is received.

No matter how much pumping I did or however long I kept my son at the breast, there was no increase in supply. I was heartbroken. Some IGT mothers make only a few soul-crushing ounces a day. I am lucky that I only needed to supplement with 3 to 10 ounces of formula per day. Perhaps because my IGT was less severe, I was able to keep my son at the breast during that first year. Using an at-breast supplementer for the formula was a huge help in keeping him nursing while he received the extra nutrition that he needed. Little did I know that once he got the hang of nursing, he had no intention of giving it up, no matter how little milk was available!

Despite having IGT, I was able to continue nursing my son, and as the days and months rolled along, continuing to nurse helped us to heal those initial wounds from him being unable to breastfeed exclusively. As a toddler, his demand finally met with my supply! For 18 months, we were just a regular breastfeeding dyad. He nursed several times a day and at naps and bedtime, but I was able to put limits on what was convenient for me *("We do not nurse at Home Depot!").* Then, I got pregnant, and my son kept nursing.

If you are nursing a 3-year-old, chances are that you may also be nursing someone else (or getting ready to). The standard advice for tandem-nursing mothers is that while your supply may drop, you will easily make enough for two when the new baby arrives, but as a mother with IGT, I was nearly certain that this advice would not apply to me, and I felt alone in my concerns of whether or not I would be able to feed both of my babies. Part of me wanted to keep nursing to ease my son's transition into life with a sibling, but part of me hoped that he would self-wean so that I would not have to worry about forcibly weaning him if it turned out I did not have enough milk for two.

My supply did drop during my pregnancy, but he kept nursing occasionally through the day and always at night. I thought for sure that he would wean during my pregnancy, given that my supply was low in the first place. However, as he approached 3 and my belly swelled, the nursing never stopped.

When my daughter arrived, I did my best as an IGT mom: I pumped, I took supplements, and we weighed her frequently to see that she was gaining. Things looked good for a few days. My son nursed at bedtime after she had eaten, and once or twice during the day for a minute or two. He seemed amenable to waiting until she was done, but then her weight dropped. We supplemented again, and my son's nursing sessions were forcibly dropped to only one. This was a very abrupt change for him. I was denying him access to me and my milk, which he had never experienced before.

Given that the baby's needs were paramount, we reduced his nursing sessions as gently as possible. During the day, I would ask him to let his sister go first and hope that he would forget by the time she was done, and this worked pretty effectively. Three-year-olds are easily distracted! At bedtime, I offered him an almost empty breast to make sure that she had gotten what she needed. As was probably the pattern for our entire nursing relationship, it did not seem to matter that there was very little *"me-me milk"* there. It mattered more to him that he got to spend any time at the breast at all.

Reducing his daytime sessions was fairly easy with substitution (a glass of milk or water), delay, and distraction, but night weaning was rough. At 3, he generally nursed once in the middle of the night and again in the morning, but both of those sessions had to stop. During the night, he slept in another room with his dad, but I could still hear him wake and ask to nurse through the wall. He cried and cried, and it broke my heart. Here I was again, unable to breastfeed either of them as much as we wanted. It took several days of tears before I was able to accept that while things were not going to be perfect, I could still have a long-term nursing relationship with both of them. Perhaps he would be able to self-wean when he was ready, and maybe his sister would be a nursing preschooler as well!

A few weeks later, my daughter was back to exclusively breast-feeding! Although he asked several times at first, we did not increase my son's nursing sessions in order to ensure that my daughter would get enough to eat as her appetite grew. Occasionally, he pretended to nurse during the day, but after the first three months or so, he seemed to be at peace with nursing only once at bedtime. If anything, that is the benefit of nursing a preschooler: he understands that his sister has to breastfeed and that she does not eat food like he does. This capacity for rational thinking helped us immensely during this transition.

As my son's fourth birthday approaches, he is still adamant about a bedtime nursing session, and it is easy for me to offer a mostly empty breast to fill that need. Sometimes, he nurses only for a few minutes, and other nights, it is closer to 15 minutes. Many times, I have to put limits on the length of that nursing session if his sister has bitten me or if I am just unable to stand any more nursing after putting two nurslings to bed. I feel strongly that when he is ready, he will fall asleep on his own, but given that the evening feed is often the last one to go, I have prepared myself to nurse him for the foreseeable future. Thankfully, nursing just once a day is very doable!

I often hear that breastfeeding is more than just milk, and my nursing relationship with my preschooler is a testament to that. Clearly, he receives more than just calories from nursing, and it is very important to me that I meet those emotional needs until he is ready to move on. IGT has thrown a few hurdles into that plan as I try to balance his needs with his sister's very real caloric needs during her first year. The problem with IGT is that even with all this demand that I have, my supply does not respond commensurately. Neither of my children can understand what IGT means and the limits that it has put on the amount of milk that I have for them. Instead, they focus only on the fact that Mama has milk, which, as my son says, makes them *"grow big and strong!"*

"Now, more than three years into this journey, when I look down into my daughter's peaceful face after she has fallen asleep at my breast, her long limbs draped across my body in true and blissful surrender, I know that this has all been worth all the energy I have poured into it. I know that my baby girl continues to need my milk in order to grow and thrive, even with autism."

—Brenda Lory

Healing through Breast Milk

Kimberly, Vine Grove, Kentucky

As a mother of a child with special needs, I sometimes feel alone. I have met other moms whose children have the same condition as my child, but I have yet to meet anyone who takes the same approach that I take.

My son is 4 and still receives breast milk daily. I consider it to be a vital part of his healing process. He no longer nurses, so I express my milk for him. We all know that feeding expressed breast milk is not the same as breastfeeding, so I sometimes feel left out of the breastfeeding world too. So, how did I get to the point of hand-expressing several times a day for a 4-year-old? Here is my story.

In June 2009, I gave birth to my first child, a son. He was beautiful and perfect, and I was in love. Breastfeeding was easy for both of us, and we had a smooth nursing relationship for a year. Just after his first birthday, I became pregnant again, and he continued to nurse throughout my pregnancy until the milk disappeared. He weaned himself when he was 20 months old, just three weeks before his sister was born.

After my daughter was born and the milk started flowing, I offered to let him nurse again. He tried a few times but seemed to have forgotten how. He eventually gave up and didn't try again. During the first year of my daughter's life, I pumped and donated nearly 1,000 ounces of milk. My son received some of my pumped milk but not much. I thought that younger babies needed it more than he did. I just accepted that this phase of our relationship was over and he no longer needed it, but I was wrong. He did need it, and our breastfeeding journey had just begun.

I knew that there was something different about my son, something that wasn't quite right, but for the longest time, I didn't know what it was. He didn't talk, he stopped making eye contact, and he didn't play. He lost many skills that he had as a young toddler. Then, in February 2012, when he was 2 years 8 months old, he was diagnosed with autism. It had been exactly a year since he had weaned, a year in which he had regressed in every developmental area. My first thought was that he needed my milk again. He needed it for his brain development, he needed it to heal the intestinal issues that came along with his autism, and he needed it to strengthen his weakened immune system.

After his diagnosis, the first thing that I did was change his diet and mine, and I started expressing milk for him every day. We both started on a gluten-free organic diet. Gluten, a protein found in many grains, can cause digestive problems for many people, especially people with autism. Going gluten-free can help many people with autism. Casein, a milk protein, can also cause some of the same problems as gluten, so many people with autism are both gluten and casein-free. Fortunately, the casein in human milk is very easily digested and does not cause any of the problems caused by the casein in the milk of other species.

Giving up some of my favorite foods was difficult, but it was so worth it when I saw such a huge improvement in my son's ability to connect with the world around him. Receiving breast milk again strengthened his immune system and healed the digestive issues he had been having.

He stopped getting sick, and he stopped having chronic diarrhea. Within a week, he started making eye contact and interacting with me again, and he started trying to talk. It was like a miracle! I don't know what made the most difference: removing gluten, eating exclusively organic, or receiving milk again. It was probably a combination of all three, but I believe that the milk made the biggest difference.

Since then, I have met other families who have said their children regressed into autism soon after weaning, but I have yet to meet anyone who has chosen to express milk for their autistic child after weaning. However, I have met families who gave their autistic children raw cow, goat, or camel milk because they believed that the raw milk improved many of their children's symptoms. I am just so thankful that I have free, fresh, raw human milk for my son. I am so thankful for my ability to lactate, and I know that it has helped him in ways that nothing else can.

Most breastfeeding mothers can understand the feeling of empowerment that they get from watching their infant grow and thrive on their milk alone. Imagine that feeling times a million over when that same milk helps to heal a child from a mysterious disorder that has no cure and no known cause. I am able to do something to help my child that no doctor in the world can do. Of course, he still has autism, but it is not nearly as severe as it was the day he was diagnosed. In a year, he moved from the severe to the mild end of the spectrum.

We have implemented other interventions during that year, including applied behavioral analysis (ABA) therapy five days a week. The therapy has helped, but I know my milk has helped even more. The essential fatty acids and other nutrients in the milk have worked within his body to improve his cognitive abilities beyond anything I ever thought possible.

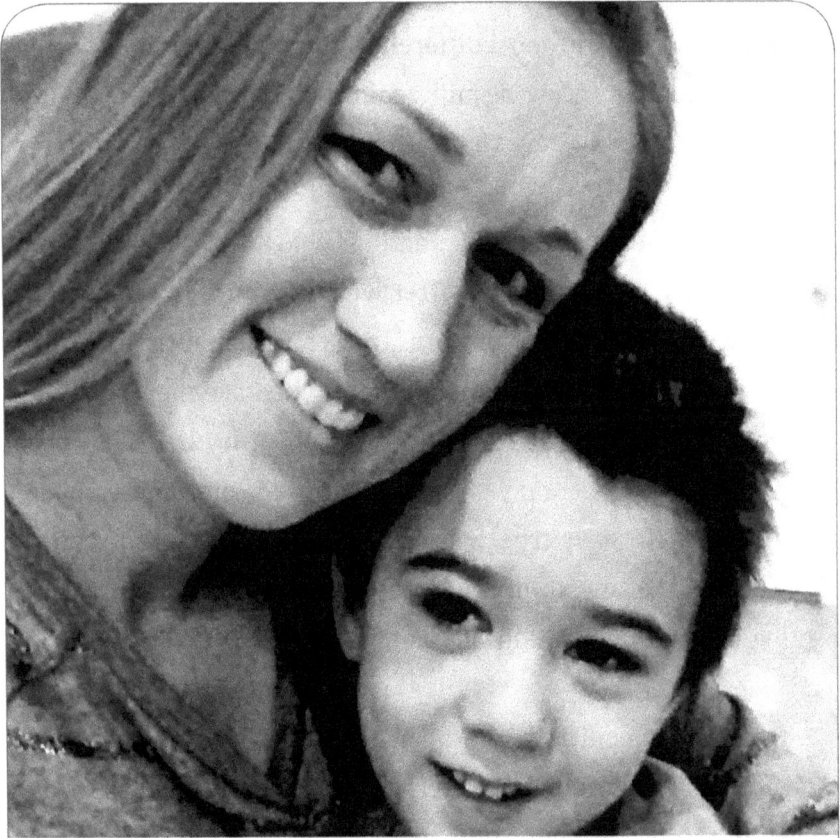

Kimberly and her son Kazim enjoying a cuddle.

His ABA therapist has been working with autistic children for 15 years, and he says he has never seen a child progress as rapidly as my son has. I give the credit to my magic milk! The therapist thought I was a little weird at first when I sent my son to therapy with a sippy cup of breast milk every day, but he has always respectfully accepted it.

I initially felt a little awkward about telling people that my son still drinks my milk at age 4, but now I'm proud of it. I work hard to express milk for him several times each day, and the hard work has paid off. I have found that most people are supportive and accepting of it, especially when I explain the reason for it.

I'm also still nursing my daughter, who is now nearly 3 years old. She will continue to nurse for as long as she wants, and I will continue to express milk for my son as long as the milk keeps flowing.

Challenging and Changing My Own Philosophy
Melanie Good Meyers, Pittsburgh, Pennsylvania

In 2001, when I became pregnant with my first child, I had no intentions of breastfeeding. I viewed breastfeeding as antiquated and sexist. I firmly believed that all childcare duties should be evenly split between mom and dad, including infant feeding. I also believed that science and technology had progressed enough that by now, surely, formula was just as good as breast milk.

When my mother learned that I was not planning to breastfeed, she was surprised and concerned. She had already been trying to convince me of the merits of natural childbirth.

I regarded her as quite the martyr for refusing pain medications when I was born, and her explanation that she did not want her baby to arrive into the world all drugged did not seem to make any sense to me. I said, *"Mom, I don't remember being born, but you sure remember giving birth. Why would you care if I was drugged if I have no recollection of it when you could have spared yourself pain?"*

However, with the topic of breastfeeding, she seemed much more insistent that I reconsider. She had breastfed me and my sister in the 1970s when breastfeeding rates were very low. She said that it was much healthier for the baby. When I contended that formula was just as good, she said that most definitely was not the case. I told her that a lot had probably changed since the 70s and that I was sure formula had been perfected since that time. She pleaded with me to do some research before I made a final decision.

I loved going to the book store anyway and knew that I could use a book that would help prepare me for childbirth, so I considered her idea of getting more information. I browsed the section on maternity and automatically rejected any titles that appeared to have an agenda to me. If it was entitled *Natural Childbirth* or *Birth without Medication* or anything like that, I did not even consider it. Then I stumbled on an unassuming title, *The Birth Book* by William and Martha Sears. I had no idea who the authors were (little did I know that they promoted an attachment parenting style), but the title seemed neutral, and the book did seem to have some chapters about medication in childbirth and infant feeding choices, so I hastily decided that it seemed balanced enough and bought it.

That book changed my entire perspective! Reading it, along with a book that a parent of one of my students had lent me, made a huge difference in my birth and parenting decisions. I realized how wrong I had been about formula, and I told my mother that she had been right. I quit seeing my very large and medicalized practice of obstetricians and switched to a small practice of certified nurse midwives. I gave birth to my first mostly naturally and breastfed her on demand. I attended my first La Leche League meeting when she was a month old and developed a network of like-minded nursing moms.

We encountered few problems in our breastfeeding relationship until she was 14 months old and I learned that I was pregnant with her sister. My milk supply dropped seemingly overnight. Even though I historically had suffered from oversupply, within weeks, I was producing only a precious few drops. Furthermore, it was becoming very uncomfortable to breastfeed. My daughter clearly did not want to wean. She continued to nurse many times during the day and night, but with the precipitous drop in my supply and her lack of sippy-cup mastery (she'd never taken a bottle either), she became dehydrated and constipated. We quickly had to get her drinking adequately from a cup, and she soon learned to complement her fluid intake from other sources. However, I was still pretty miserable. Each nursing session felt like sandpaper on my nipples, and the ones in the middle of the night were the worst because the irritation would wake me up fully. In the past, we had mostly dream-nursed without either of us fully awakening in our family bed. Now, every morning, I would feel like a zombie from all of the disruption to my sleep and also so touched out that daytime nursing, with the accompanying irritation, felt like torture.

So, I made the choice to night-wean my toddler. I bought the book *Adventures in Tandem Nursing* by Hilary Flower, which was full of ideas and encouragement on nursing through pregnancy and tandem nursing. We gently weaned her at night over the course of about a month, with her daddy taking over the nighttime comforting and offering her a sippy cup of water if she was thirsty. It was a bit of a tricky transition, but once I could get a full night's sleep, it was easier to deal with the daytime irritation with nursing. I was so glad that I made this compromise because she continued to nurse through the whole pregnancy, and we went on to tandem-nurse for another two years!

Of those two years of tandem nursing, the first few months were pretty intense. My oldest was delighted that there was finally milk again, and she nursed almost as frequently as her newborn sister.

I generally tried to have my newborn nurse first, and occasionally, I did nurse them simultaneously, but it was somewhat awkward to balance a toddler and a newborn together, so I found myself nursing them separately most of the time. Because of how frequently they were both nursing, I had a huge appetite! I remember one morning downing five smoothies for breakfast! However, I managed to maintain my vegan diet and shed my pregnancy weight at a gradual, healthy pace, and meanwhile, my daughters each gained well over 2 pounds in the first month! It was a very powerful feeling to know I had produced enough milk to help them grow so substantially.

Over the next year, though, my oldest began nursing less and less frequently. By age 2½, she wasn't nursing every day, but I still found nursing her to be of great benefit when she was learning to deal with those toddler emotions that can lead so easily to meltdowns and anytime when she was ill (although that was infrequent) or needed comfort because of a boo-boo.

Having two nurslings and having had nursing come to feel completely normalized by my regular attendance at La Leche League meetings, I quickly overcame any feelings of anxiety about nursing in public that may have still been lingering. I had no problem nursing whenever and wherever either of my daughters needed to. Nevertheless, after my older daughter turned 3, I found that we were nursing much less in public simply because her nursing frequency had dropped off so much. Eventually, when she was around 3½ years old, I noticed that sometimes two weeks would go by without her nursing, and I started thinking that maybe she had weaned, but then she would ask to nurse again, and I would always oblige. Then, shortly after my older daughter's 4th birthday, she announced that she was going to wean soon, and within a month, she said she was done with *"boosies."*

My second daughter continued to nurse, and I assumed that it would be another year or two before she weaned since she was just over 2 when her sister weaned and was still nursing every day. However, there were difficulties in my first marriage at the time that my older daughter weaned. I had returned to school to further my education, and this was one of the many sources of stress in our marriage. It was difficult to juggle my night classes with her night nursing, so I decided to gently night-wean her as I had with my oldest, assuming that it would not impact our nursing relationship that much. However, between the night weaning and the marital strife, I noticed that her nursing frequency dropped off precipitously. Perhaps part of it was also that she was following her big sister's lead, but I began trying to counteract her rapid drop-off in nursing by offering to nurse her whenever I had an opportunity. This had limited success. Mostly, she would just latch on for a minute or two and then want to run off and play. Other times, she just wasn't interested at all. Sometimes a week would go by without a nursing session.

Finally, when she was about 32 or 33 months old, I realized that it had been a long time since she had nursed, and I offered to nurse her. She seemed interested, but when she went to latch on, she didn't seem to know what to do anymore and just giggled and said she was all done with nursing. A few more times over the next year, she did randomly ask to nurse out of nowhere, but each time, she could not remember how to latch on. At one point, she got rather sad about it and wished that she hadn't stopped nursing so that she would remember how. I still am not certain which factor was most responsible for the rapid pace of her weaning, although I suspect that it was a complex combination of all of the situational factors and her own personal timetable. Whatever the reasons, she was basically weaned before her third birthday, much sooner than I had expected. I mourned the loss of our nursing relationship since it had happened much more rapidly than I had anticipated, and because my marriage had just broken up around the same time, I assumed that my nursing years were done.

However, as fate would have it, I met a wonderful man and found myself married again four years after my divorce. We were soon thrilled to be welcoming a new baby into our family. My son was born in 2011, and he took to nursing like a champ. We did struggle with recurrent thrush for the first 14 months of his life (I blame the antibiotics that I had in labor with him for group B strep), and that was frustrating. However, he was growing well and thriving the whole time. My son is now 25 months old and still nurses several times each day and a few times at night. I do not plan to night-wean him as I did with my daughters because I am fortunate to have a great supportive husband and no scheduling or other logistics to manage. I also want to wait until he is weaned before we consider whether we want any more children, so I do not anticipate any hormonal changes pushing me to night-wean either. I currently work part time, and it does not seem to interfere with our nursing relationship. My son seems quite contented to continue nursing, and I am happy to keep nursing him. I am sure that his journey toward weaning will be as individual as each of my daughters' was, and someday, I will look back fondly on these days as a memory.

Over the years, I have encountered challenges, including plugged ducts, overactive letdown, mastitis, milk blisters, and thrush, but I have always persevered because I have been determined to give my children the gift that my mother had given me all those years ago. Although I was not breastfed for as long as my children, I am eternally grateful for that gift and for my mother's encouragement for me to give that gift to my children. Now, I have an 11-year-old, a 9-year-old, and a 2-year-old who have always been very healthy and happy.

Beyond the nutritional and immunological benefits that I have given my children, I also believe that I have given them a special human bond that is simply priceless. I hope that someday I will see my grandchildren breastfed, just as my mom cherishes her breastfed grandchildren.

I would like to share a poem written by my grandmother, who passed away in 2011. She often talked about becoming a mother during the Great Depression, how she had no financial choice but to breastfeed, and how she also thought that it was the most natural thing in the world and wondered why everyone didn't breastfeed. Her parenting style is captured in this poem—apparently, she practiced attachment parenting before the term was even coined!

Motherhood poem
by Sarah A. Good

Pick me up my mother,

Hold me in your arms,

Hold me tight against your soft, warm breast.

Pick me up my darling,

Hold me in your arms,

For that's the way I like to take my rest.

Pick me up my mother,

Hold your face close to mine,

Rocking, rocking, gently to and fro.

Hold me close my mother,

Hold me in your arms,

While quietly, off to sleep I go.

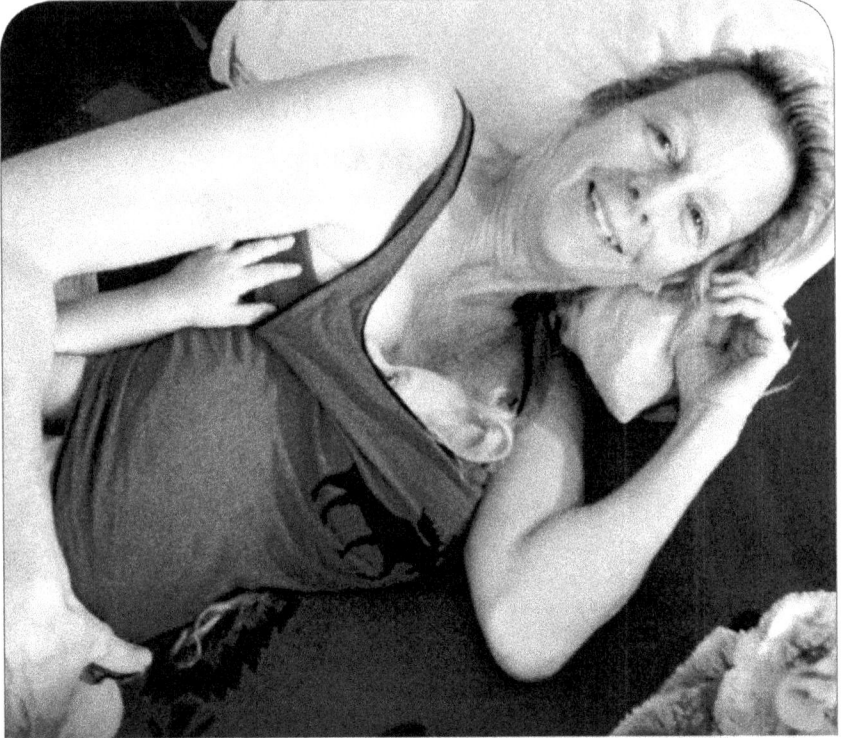

A snuggle under Mommy's shirt for Mommy's milk.

Winnie and Jo Gayler, Nokomis, Florida.

Depression, Anxiety, and Pressure to Wean
Olivia Hinebaugh, Burke, Virginia

B efore I had Callum, I had mental health concerns. At 23, I was struck suddenly with crippling panic attacks, agoraphobia, and the depression that so often goes along with these conditions. After just a year of therapy and medication, my issues were completely resolved. Thinking these things were behind me, my husband and I set out to try to conceive.

The road to Callum's birth was uncomplicated. I conceived easily. Pregnant, I felt vibrant and mentally strong. I loved every change that occurred in my body, and I longed for the breastfeeding connection that I had heard so much about. After a long but calm labor, Callum arrived peacefully and was healthy and ready to nurse.

Like any new mom, I had a few bumps in the road: sore nipples, oversupply, and overactive letdown. We stuck with it. I didn't see quitting as a choice. It never even entered my mind. I felt powerful as a nursing mother: able to comfort, feed, and nurture my child.

I got the usual spiel from the pediatrician at 4 to 6 months about introducing solids. I knew in my gut that Callum wasn't ready. In fact, his first real solid food came at about 11 months when he wolfed down the burrito I had been about to eat.

It was around his first birthday that I saw the dreaded signs of my anxiety returning. I had had a few panic attacks spread out over the months, but day to day, things were getting worse. My world began shrinking as it had before. I no longer wanted to go on little trips into Washington, DC, take public transportation, or go anywhere where I might encounter bumper-to-bumper traffic. I knew that it was time to get back into some form of treatment.

I saw my HMO-assigned therapist, who immediately told me that it was time to get back on medication. Then, I met with a psychiatrist. This was the most brutal experience to date in my few years as a mother. She agreed that, yes, it was time to start treatment with antidepressants and antianxiety medications. She said that none of these had been proven safe for breastfeeding, and she asked how old my son was.

"He just had his first birthday," I told her.

"Oh, so you can wean," she said coldly. *"Breastfeeding is only beneficial for the first year."*

"I don't know that I can. He's only just starting on solids. He still needs it to go to sleep. He still nurses every 4 hours or so."

"Well, you need to make a choice. It isn't safe to breastfeed and be on these medications. The right thing for you, and the best thing for your baby, is for you to wean and be a healthy and functional mother."

I sobbed right there in her office. She was telling me that I had failed as a mother. I had let myself get sick. I had raised a dependent kid. I was making a selfish choice to breastfeed instead of getting well. All of my stout defenses of attachment parenting flew out the window. I started questioning my deep connection with my baby, who, yes, was still a baby. Had I spoiled him? Was I a terrible mother if I didn't take him to the zoo or on the metro? Forget me quoting the World Health Organization's recommendation to breastfeed until at least the age of 2. I couldn't recall the many, many reasons that I was still nursing.

I left that appointment with an impossible decision: nurture myself or nurture my child—my beautiful, blonde-haired, breast-loving boy, whose first word was *"nun,"* his word for nursing.

I mourned for what I thought would be the end of my breastfeeding relationship for a few days. I spent countless weeping hours talking to my husband and my mother about what this psychiatrist had told me, and God bless them, they were the first to point out that maybe this psychiatrist was wrong. Surely, I was not the first woman to encounter these problems. Think of all the women with devastating postpartum depression. Surely, they didn't need to choose between weaning and medicating?

I asked my circle of mom friends and found that a surprising number of them also took antidepressants for a wide variety of reasons. It was beautiful to learn that I wasn't alone. I slowly gained back my confidence in how I had chosen to parent. If I was able to shrug when my son was 4 months old and I was told by a well-meaning doctor that I might kill Callum if he slept in bed with us, and if I had eventually let go of the pressure to rush solids, surely I could remain steadfast in my desire to nurse my toddler. It was more than a desire. I saw no way around it, at least no way that wasn't paved in trauma for both of us.

I saw another psychiatrist. Not enough can be said about how wonderful she was. There was no judgment when she heard that I was still nursing. There was nothing but reassurance for the studies that were out there. She agreed that my son didn't need to wean for me to get treatment. She showed me the statistics on all of the different antidepressants, and together, we chose one that not only had been effective for other members of my family but that was excreted only in very small amounts into breast milk. Then, she said something wonderful: it seemed like I was doing the very best that I could for my baby.

I cried in her office too. She understood and was going to help me. I had done the right thing.

As a mother, I had always listened to my gut. Callum didn't like his crib, so he slept in bed with us. I loved nursing him to sleep. He didn't take a bottle, and that was fine because we belonged together for those first two years. When he didn't seem ready for solids, I waited. He got it eventually, as I knew he would.

Now, Callum is a thriving 3-year-old, and I have another child. He has continued to nurse. It's been uncomfortable at times, and my milk dried up completely during pregnancy when I was hit with a stomach bug, but that hasn't diminished his desire to curl up with his mom and nurse. Toddlers get banged up and have emotional breakdowns, but there is still nothing that sitting in my lap and looking into my eyes and nursing won't cure.

I saw a therapist as part of my treatment who was horrified to hear that I was still nursing even though I was newly pregnant with another child. She couldn't hide her disgust and her judgment, and raised concerns about me nurturing a child at the breast and another in the womb. I never went back to her. She said what she said out of concern, but she was wrong. This time, I knew that she was wrong.

I've continued to nurse my son, through ups and downs, changes in medication, through a pregnancy and a birth, past his first, second, and third birthdays. He shows no signs of stopping. Even on days when my anxiety is at an all-time high, one thing I never worry about is nurturing and loving my sweet Callum. He may come to realize that his mama has struggles, but I don't think that he will ever doubt that I will be there for him every day. Breastfeeding is one of the ways that I show this to him.

Mental illness can be very isolating. I am eternally grateful for my support system. It was talking things through with my mother, husband, and friends that gave me the courage to continue on my path of extended breastfeeding. However, most of all, it was those moments when my whole world was calm and wonderful and it was just me and Callum, nursing, bonding, and taking care of each other.

Breastfeeding a 5-Year-Old Is Easy!
My Full-Term Breastfeeding Story (So Far)

Sarah Langford, Melbourne, Australia[10]

I have been breastfeeding every day for over five years. I have breastfed through engorgement and nipple shields. I have breastfed in my sleep and through nipple thrush. I have breastfed on planes and trains, leaning over child-safe car seats in moving vehicles, on buses, boats, and ferries, in the sea, on the sand, and on the grass. I have breastfed hanging half my body over a pram. I have breastfed at protest rallies, while baby-wearing, in the middle of giving public speeches, and while pushing another child on the swing. I have breastfed while literally rubbing shoulders with a conservative politician. I have breastfed through flashbacks to sexual abuse and taken breastfeeding breaks while getting tattoos. I have breastfed two children at a time. I have breastfed friends' children. I have expressed my breast milk and sent it to three different babies in need. I have used expressed breast milk to treat my children's ear infections and my partner's colds and flus. I have breastfed during childbirth. I have breastfed while attending other babies' births. I have breastfed through pregnancy twice and juggled three breast-feeding children.

Honestly, the older they get, the easier they are to breastfeed. This is what my journey with my eldest has taught me. Deep down, I never expected to be successful at breastfeeding. With each passing month, I have been amazed that I am still doing it, that my body is

---

10   This story was adapted from a blog post originally published on Sarah's blog, *Ilithia Inspired*, on June 8, 2013, which can be found at http://www.ilithyiainspired.com/2013/06/breast-feeding-5-year-old-is-easy.html, along with links to more of Sarah's articles on breastfeeding.

capable, and that my daughter is growing. I could hardly believe my eyes, and this is part of the reason that we have such a rich catalog of breastfeeding photos of the two of us: I believed that it couldn't last and that I needed to record and preserve all that I could.

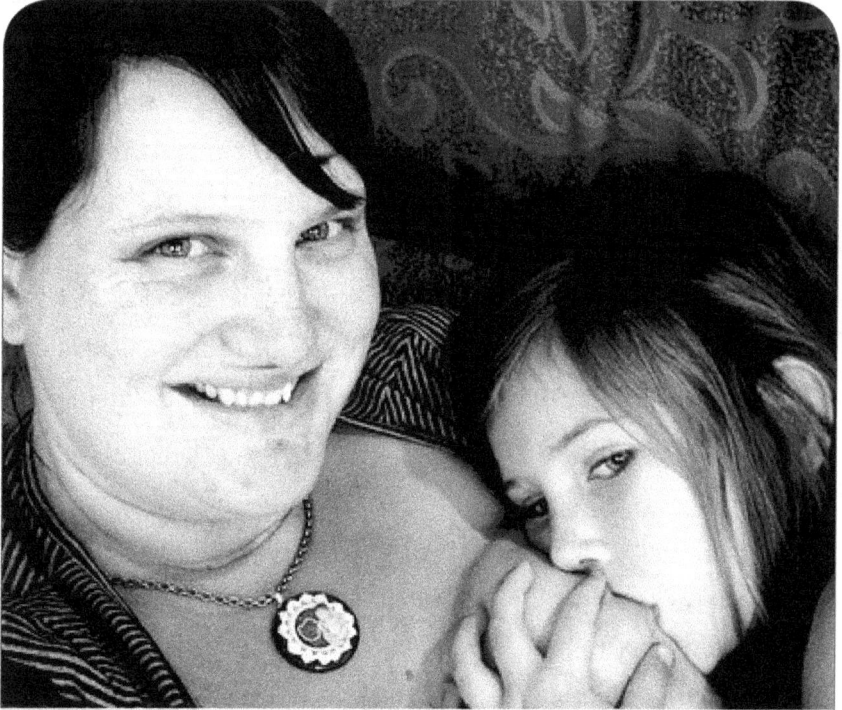

Sarah and Harriet.

I had more fears about learning to breastfeed than I did about the pain of childbirth. My anxiety led to poor planning, and in my birth plan, I gave permission to my doulas to be hands-on and overly involved in establishing breastfeeding. As they touched my body in that first hour and handled me and my baby, although they were well-meaning, I became despondent and felt myself leave my body. This confirmed for me that I didn't know what to do and that

I wouldn't be able to breastfeed. A couple of days later, when I was engorged, one of my doulas breastfed Harriet and said that she was starving and I didn't know it. At the time, I felt like I could die and it wouldn't matter: I was useless, and anyone else with breast milk could feed my daughter better than I could. However, I was grateful that she didn't push artificial milk and bottles onto us.

I had serious body-image issues when it came to my breasts. These were linked to my adolescent experiences of sexual abuse. When I started leaking colostrum halfway through my first pregnancy, it triggered those memories, and I reacted with tears, fears, and disgust. While I worked through some of these issues during pregnancy, flashbacks to sexual abuse were a reality during those early breastfeeding days.

During nighttime feeds, I had to have the light on and breathe through my reactive feelings of repulsion, during which it felt like my skin was crawling. It was very hard to separate the present breastfeeding moment from memories of my abuser touching my breasts. However, with time and support, I was able to work through it, and it rarely happens now, years later.

Harriet and I overcame engorgement, big breasts and little nipples, and misguided advice from a breastfeeding counselor that led us to unnecessarily using nipple shields and spending eight weeks weaning ourselves off them.

Finally, at about the 10-week mark, everything finally fell into place, and I found myself wandering around my partner's office, breastfeeding my baby without shields, chatting to people as I walked and fed. From there, breastfeeding flowed for Harriet and me.

I was committed to breastfeeding and working through challenges because I wanted to do everything in my power to meet my child's needs. Breast milk is every child's birthright, and the health of children who miss out on breastfeeding is compromised, so I never considered weaning an option. I found that minor breastfeeding challenges presented themselves every now and again and often coincided with developmental milestones for my growing girl. These included some brief nipple sensitivity with the return of my menstrual cycle, sudden drops in the number of feeds and the amount of time that she spent at the breast, and the reverse—sudden increases.

The biggest challenge we've had since those newborn days has been her changing latch. As she grows, her face changes, as do her mouth and her teeth. Every now and again, her latch will become uncomfortable for me for a period. We work through it with shorter feeds and by readjusting the latch.

Even as a 2-year-old, she was very understanding and would come off the breast for a moment, open her mouth wide, poke her tongue out a little, and reattach herself. This was how we managed to continue to breastfeed, including throughout the night, through my second pregnancy. At the time of this writing, Harriet and I are feeding through a pregnancy for a second time.

Adjusting to sharing my breasts with her newborn sister was challenging for Harriet at times. I'm not sure how much of that was really about breastfeeding, though. I think that any 2-year-old struggles with the arrival of a new sibling. There were some intense tantrums in the first six weeks of her sister's life. One such tantrum was so loud that the police showed up at our door after someone reported that a child was being abused at our address! The police took one look at me feeding the newborn on the couch and asked how old Harriet was. By the time they arrived, she had moved through her emotions and was happily playing naked. She greeted the police at the door enthusiastically with *"Pizza?"* The police then apologized for intruding and assured me that they understood our parenting predicament.

The World Health Organization breastfeeding recommendations always gave me comfort, as did knowing that the average global weaning age is 4 years. I had expected that Harriet would wean at 3, but she was still as enthusiastic about *"boobee"* as she'd ever been. On her fourth birthday, I was amazed to discover that we were still at it. I was sure she'd wean at 4. Her feeding definitely dropped a lot during that year, but then we were at her fifth birthday and still going.

When she was 4, I started to become self-conscious about breast-feeding Harriet in public. While during the first four years of breast-feeding, I had felt confident and responded to public criticism with scientific facts, in that fifth year, I was starting to feel worn down by social attitudes and did not want to deal with them anymore.

I felt conflicted. On the one hand, I remained committed to supporting my daughter in determining her own time frame for weaning and knew that all of the comfort and nutrition that she was continuing to receive from breastfeeding was ensuring her optimal physical, emotional, and psychological development. On the other hand, I was afraid that the only memories she would have of breastfeeding would be of rude looks and discouraging comments from strangers if we continued to nurse whenever and wherever she needed. For the first time in our breastfeeding relationship, I started using blankets to cover up and talking to Harriet about breastfeeding *"safe places,"* such as at home and at trusted friends' houses, and not so much at bus stops and shopping centers anymore. I explained that I wanted boobee to always be a happy time for her and never rushed, and this was why we were going to wait to feed sometimes.

I tried to work through my issues because ultimately it wasn't fair to Harriet. On occasion, I would still oblige her when she asked to feed in public; it was rare that she did, anyway. However, increasingly, my answer was, *"Not right now, honey,"* or *"When we get home?"* She fed less; she was very understanding. Yet, there I was, five years down the track, making choices that I wasn't comfortable with, compromising Harriet's breastfeeding journey because of social attitudes. This was something that I would never have stood for even two years before because nothing should be more important to me as a mother than my child's well-being. However, *"lactophobia"* had finally infected me, and I was prioritizing the ignorant prejudices of strangers above my child's needs.

Interestingly, most of the public criticism that I've received while breastfeeding happened before my children were 2. I suspect that the bigger she got, the more confusing her breastfeeding was to strangers, and they were too shocked to say anything. But when she was little, there were a few awkward moments where strangers felt that they needed to share their ignorance with me. In particular, I remember the racist at a bus stop who asked where I came from. When I replied in my most occa accent *"Oss-traaaaayl-yah,"* she replied, *"And you do that there, do you?!"* gesturing to my *"grotesque"* breastfeeding.

In the earlier days, when I faced a breastfeeding challenge, I would go to my local Australian Breastfeeding Association group, ring the helpline, or talk to friends for support. However, the longer we feed, the less support there is to be found. It's rare to find a breastfeeding counselor who has had firsthand experience with breastfeeding a 5-year-old. Most of Harriet's breastfed peers have weaned, although if she knows this, it doesn't bother her. Thankfully, the challenges of feeding an older child are not life-threatening like in those early days when you worry about supply and ensuring that baby is getting enough milk. Even the discomfort and latch issues are easily resolved between the two of us now that she's older. The challenges now are external to our breastfeeding relationship: they're cultural.

Something that has helped a lot has been reading Ann Sinnott's book, *Breastfeeding Older Children*. Reading this book has gone a long way in normalizing full-term breastfeeding for me. When I read about other mother's experiences with breastfeeding children older than 5, I was relieved to learn that Harriet and I are not the only ones. I was particularly comforted by reading Sinnott's own journey of working through similar issues when feeding her 6-year-old:

> *"A process of querying and challenging my own*
> *feelings was set in train, and finally I understood*

that my reactions were founded on nothing more than cultural assumptions. Though there may be exceptions, it now seems to me that there is the strongest likelihood that there are valid, non-pathologic, reasons for the continuance of the intermittent feeding patterns that seem to typify the upper ages."

She cites a few legitimate reasons that children should want to continue breastfeeding, including the following: it's a stressful world, the human immune system doesn't mature until a child is 7, and science is slowly learning that breast milk is medicine.

Sinnot argues that in a world where adults are seeking breast milk to treat cancer and science is trying to recreate breast milk to treat cancer and digestive conditions, it really isn't fair to expect young children to go without.

Research on the natural weaning time frames found in traditional societies and in primates has also reassured me that we're on the right track. One researcher found a link between animal weaning and the time that they cut their first permanent molars, which for humans happens at around 5 or 6 years of age.[11] Another study suggested that the link between weaning age and sexual maturity in primates indicates that the normal weaning age for humans would be 6 or 7 years of age.

Whatever the biological norm and whatever the reasons, Harriet expresses a need to continue breastfeeding. Continuing has always

11   *A Natural Age of Weaning,* by Katherine Dettwyler, which can be found at http:// http://www.whale.to/a/dettwyler.html.

felt right to me, while anything that encourages weaning before the desire comes from Harriet has always made me uncomfortable.

When you remove the cultural taboo around breastfeeding older children, there really isn't a reason to forcibly wean a happily feeding child. Breastfeeding a 5-year-old is easy! We face fewer challenges now than we did in the first, second, or third year of breastfeeding. She consumes other foods and drinks water like a champ. Most of the time, she seeks other forms of comfort, such as arms to hold her and ears to listen. She's a confident, healthy, and happy kid with a great sense of humor, who loves her independence and being a social butterfly. Occasionally, she prefers the comfort of suckling at her mother's breast and the delicious taste of breast milk.

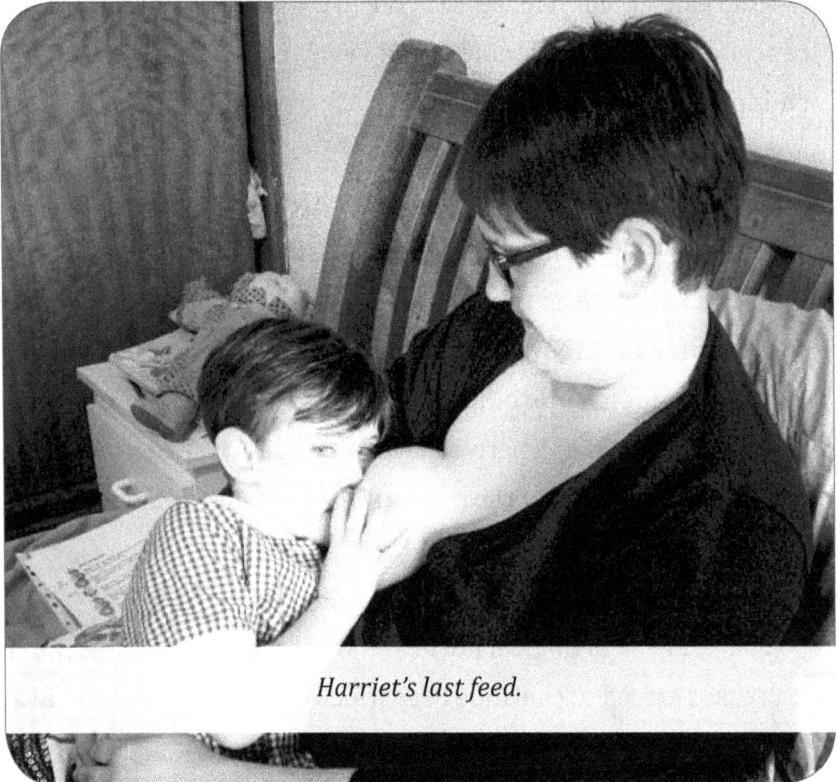

Harriet's last feed.

Postscript

At age 5 years 8 months, Harried decided to have her final breast-feed. We celebrated the end of an era with a small party, a couple of friends, and the cake of her choice—Barbie! She helped bake her special weaning cake, and we did some fingernail and toenail painting.

I am now breastfeeding only a 3-year-old and a 6-month-old. It's good to be down to two nurslings!

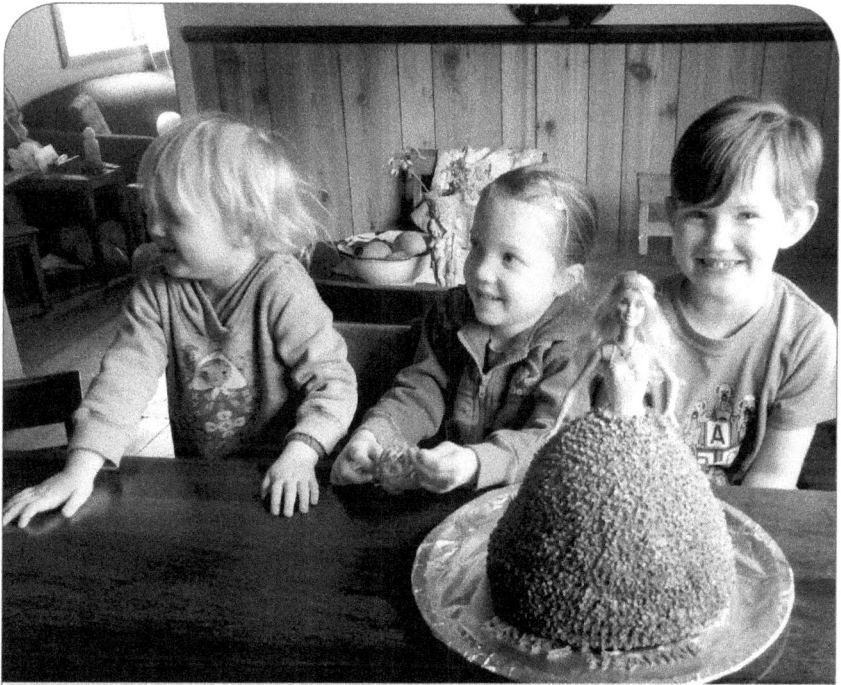

Harriet, her sister, and a friend with her weaning cake.

Breastfeeding through Travels and Troubles[12]
Joanne MacKenzie, Bellingham, Washington

I tried to breastfeed my first two daughters, who were born in Detroit, Michigan, in 1961 and 1962. My nipples cracked and bled, and it was too painful, so I gave up.

In 1966, we moved to central coastal California. In 1968, I divorced my first husband. I also met my soon-to-be second husband, and we moved to the San Francisco Bay area.

When my mother learned that I was pregnant again, she asked me if I was going to try breastfeeding again, and when I said yes, her response was, *"Well, you had better toughen up your nipples then."* I was amazed and hurt. Her tone of voice and facial expression convinced me that she had known this little bit of wisdom in 1961 and 1962 but had chosen to withhold the information.

There were many changes in the culture between the early 1960s and the 1970s, especially on the West coast. Natural childbirth and La Leche League were now available to provide support for women who chose *"alternative"* ways to give birth and nurture their babies. In 1970, my youngest daughter was born in San Francisco with the Lamaze method of natural childbirth and with my husband present in the delivery room. She was breastfed from birth and slept with us in the family bed. When she awoke at night, she squirmed around until she found a nipple and went back to sleep. She didn't wake my husband, and I was roused only enough to assist her.

When she was 6 months old, we all moved to North Africa, where my husband was employed by an American company, along with six other programmers, to create a computer system that would unify all of the various systems that the Algerian government had inherited after it nationalized the oil industry at the end of the Algerian war with France in the early 1960s.

We arrived in Algiers at 10 p.m. after having spent an entire day in the airport in Paris waiting for an available Air Algerie flight. Our little travel group consisted of my husband, myself, a 6-year-old, a 9-year-old, a 6-month-old baby, a dog in a crate, six suitcases, and a baby buggy filled with books. It took two cabs to get from the airport to the hotel St. George, where we were told that a room would be available for us. The concierge there told us that they were all booked and that we would have to get back in the taxis and drive 60 kilometers to another hotel, where they might be able to accommodate us. Of course, all of these arrangements were communicated in French, which neither my husband or myself could speak well enough.

Fortunately, on our way out, we ran into the man who had hired my husband, an American who was fluent in French, and he straightened everything out. By midnight, we were all tucked into our suite, the very one that had been occupied by General Eisenhower during World War II.

That was my introduction to how necessary it would be that I continue breastfeeding as long as possible. There was no reliable fresh milk supply. There was no dairy industry in Algeria. The country grew and exported grapes for wine, citrus fruit, avocados, and dates to feed European countries. The best of everything was shipped elsewhere. Milk was flown into the country every morning from France, delivered to all the neighborhood stores, and kept in crates on the floor beside the refrigerator, which was filled with Coke and Fanta orange soda. There was only one self-serve, government-run grocery store for at least 100 miles. Food was purchased at the open-air market in the center of Algiers or at the nearest neighborhood store, where one had to request by name and sometimes by brand name in French everything that one wanted to buy. There was no TV and no visible advertising to give one a clue about what was available.

The baby food that I was able to find was loaded with sugar, even the baby cereals. When my daughter began eating solid food, she started with mashed banana. I eventually found some jars of baby food that didn't have sugar added, so she had pureed meat mixed with banana and pureed peas mixed with banana. When there was fruit grown in Algeria available, the government stopped importing bananas; it had something to do with the balance of payments.

By necessity, I continued to breastfeed my daughter. We traveled to Europe several times, back to the United States for a month, and then back to Algiers.

I traveled by myself once with my daughter from London to Heidelberg to meet a friend. The plane had to land in Frankfurt, and a mob of very tall Germans gathered around the ticket counters trying to get flights to their final destinations. I am 5 feet 2 inches tall. I didn't have a chance, so I climbed up on a window sill, held my ticket up in the air, and breastfed my daughter. It took about 2 minutes for an airline agent to notice me and come running over to get my ticket and get me on the next flight to Heidelberg.

Breastfeeding was a necessity for many reasons. It was so easy and gave me incredible freedom from having to drag around bottles and formula. I simply could not have had this great adventure if I hadn't been nursing my child. Yes, I sometimes was teased. My daughter was referred to as my *"barnacle"* because she was always attached to me. With the judicious use of a scarf, I could feed her anywhere.

She was a delightfully happy, outgoing child who charmed people in every country that we visited.

When we returned to the United States in December of 1973, she was 3 years 4 months old. My family, whom we stopped to visit on the way back to California, asked, with disapproval in their voices, how long I was going to continue to breastfeed her. My answer was until she started school or maybe longer.

In California, I didn't encounter any disapproval. When we moved into a bedroom in a shared house, we got a mattress for our daughter to sleep on in the same room with us. My older children were with their father in southern California at that time, and we were looking for a house big enough to contain my two children, my husband's two children, and our daughter.

She always nursed at bedtime. She had never fallen asleep without being nursed. I would get into bed with her and feed her. When she fell asleep, I would get up and go to the other bed. If she awoke in the night, she would come and find me. However, because she was able to be more independent, go to nursery school, and play with neighborhood kids, she nursed less often. She had stopped napping when she was 6 months old, so feeding took place in the morning, if she hurt herself, and at bedtime. Less nursing meant less milk. At 4½, she would only occasionally want to nurse and then only for a minute or two. Weaning was a natural process, all about demand and supply. The demand decreased and so did the supply. It eventually ran out.

After our return to the United States, her father and I separated. In one week, our household went from one with two parents and five children to one with one parent and two children, and soon just one parent and one child. My oldest went off to the University of California, Berkeley, my husband's two moved with him to a different house, and my middle daughter moved out a year later. I am absolutely convinced that my youngest daughter's prolonged breastfeeding and place in the family bed gave her the resilience necessary to weather the painful breakup of our family. I was also fortunate that I didn't have to go back to work after she was born and that I wasn't living near my family of origin, which wasn't supportive of extended breastfeeding.

Today, my daughter is 42 years old, and she doesn't have a mean bone in her body. She is able to be strong and kind at the same time. I have met only one other young adult who shared some of those same qualities of openness, kindness, and gentle honesty. I learned from his mother when I met her that this child too had been breastfeed until he was 4½ and had always slept in the same bed with his parents when he was a baby and a toddler.

Chapter 6

When the End Finally Arrives

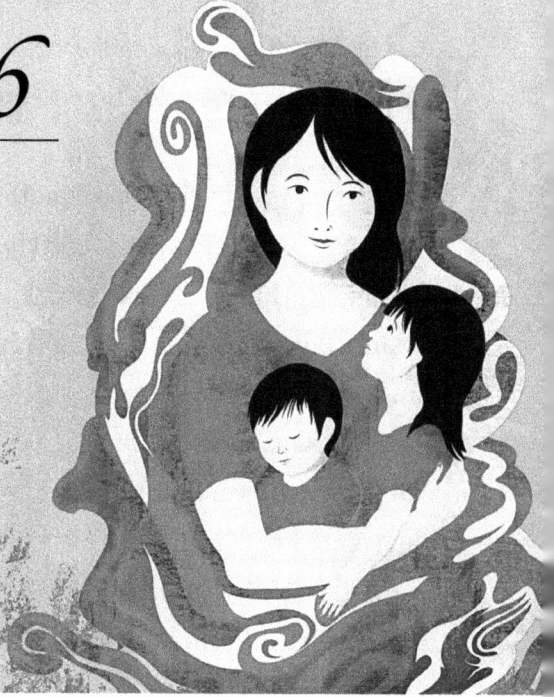

*W*eaning is the word on everyone's mind when they think of breastfeeding, especially when they talk about breastfeeding kids that can walk, talk, and sometimes roller-skate and ride a bike. However, weaning actually starts any time a child has anything other than his mother's milk. It is and has always been meant to be a slow and gradual process, although this is not always how it plays out. In this chapter, you will read about weaning as it pertains to the end of breastfeeding for a child who has been nursing for at least three years. There is no right time or right age. There is always a unique balance, ideally determined by mother and child together, that works for each nursing pair.

A Rocky Start That Ended Smoothly
Carla Parry, Lakeland, Florida

Some might say my son's weaning began at four days when he needed formula because of weight loss and a high jaundice level. We had quite the rocky, unexpected start to nursing.

You see, I was a seasoned mother with two failed breastfeeding attempts and a long list of initials that should have made it easy. I am an International Board Certified Lactation Consultant. I had 10 years of experience when my son was born and detailed plans for an easy, long-term nursing relationship. Despite our initial difficulties, I made up my mind that I would protect my milk supply and do whatever I could to encourage and allow him to nurse as long as he wanted to. This meant very little time away. I had to return to work unexpectedly when he was 4 months old. I pumped at work until he was 2 years old so that he wouldn't stop nursing because of a lack of milk.

I wasn't away from my son overnight until he was 3 years old. I told myself that I wouldn't be sad if he didn't want to nurse on my return from my three nights away, but I did pump a few times each day while I was gone (in Vegas no less!). On my return home, the first thing he asked for was *"milktaplease,"* his word for nursing. I was delighted and relieved that my time away had not been the catalyst for him weaning. We went away to Vegas again the following year when he was 4 years 4 months old. Surely, I thought, he will be done with nursing now. He was down to morning and nighttime only, but that was not to be the end. That night at bedtime on the day of our return, he asked to nurse. This time, I didn't pump, or rather couldn't express a drop, while we were away, and when I asked him if there was still milk for him, he said yes. The next six months found him requesting to nurse to sleep every night but slowly dropping the morning nursings. Those sweet morning nursings, just me and him in the chair, snuggled under a blanket. I would kiss his head and look at his long limbs, which were changing from those of a baby to those of a young boy. These are some of the sweetest moments of his weaning, and I will treasure them.

By his fifth birthday in June, he would occasionally fall asleep without nursing while I rubbed his back. On the nights that he would ask to nurse, I would tell him *"Only a minute,"* and most times, he would be happy to let go, roll over, and go to sleep. At this point, I was getting pressure from his father to wean and not for the first time in five years. My husband asked me around the one year mark, at 18 months, and then again at 2 years. Then, he gave up for a bit. My husband, seeing Ashton go to preschool at 3 and interact with other children and watching how smart and independent Ashton was, paved the way for our continued nursing without many questions. Plus, in the back of his mind, he thought the end was coming any day. Around this five year mark, he was rather insistent that a 5-year-old that was nursing would talk about it, maybe at school, and that might raise some eyebrows.

About October, my son announced, *"I'm done with milktaplease. I keep forgetting about it."* Part of me was glad that he was making the decision to stop on his own, and the emotional part of me scrambled to try to remember the last time that he had nursed and etch it in my brain. I quickly wrote down the last time he had nursed and what he had said and dated it. That night, he asked to nurse again! Then, he went five days without asking. Then, he nursed again. He went seven days without nursing before he asked again. Then, he went another 10 days and asked again for the last time. I was happy! I was happy that his weaning had not been untimely or because of some silly mistake. I was happy that he was not sad about it. I was happy because I also got to experience the joys of nursing a toddler, a preschooler, and a grade schooler. I was happy because I had laid down a foundation of physical and emotional health that I had been unable to do for my other children, despite our very rocky start. There were no tears on my part or his. I had no regrets.

Today, he is 6 years 5 months old. It has been almost exactly one year since his weaning day. He talks about nursing occasionally and has a fondness for snuggling against my breast when he is still for a moment. He is healthy, independent, and creative and a social butterfly! He weighs over 60 pounds and is very tall. Sometimes, I look at him and can't believe that he found comfort in my breast just a year ago. I hope that Ashton's self-weaning helps him to be supportive of his own children's nursing one day. I hope that my daughters (who are 22 and 21 years old) are impacted positively by their brother's nursing beyond the expected societal norm, even though they both had untimely weanings.

My hope in telling Ashton's weaning story is that other moms who may get off to a rocky start with breastfeeding or need supplementation will know that full-term nursing or child-led weaning is still possible.

Mother-Led, Child-Honoring Weaning
Lauren Wayne, Seattle, Washington

There's something to be said for a gentle, child-honoring weaning, even if it's mama-led. I'd wanted to let my older son set the terms for his own weaning, but eventually, I stepped in to guide us both to a peaceful, if somewhat bittersweet conclusion to our five years of breastfeeding.

After a rough early start in the hospital, I was happy that my nursing relationship with my firstborn, Mikko, continued smoothly on...and on. The birthdays passed—the first, second, and third—and we were still going strong. There was no reason to stop. He was obviously getting both physical and emotional benefits from continuing to breastfeed, and I had no objections. I liked that we had such a strong and special bond and that I was able to nourish him in this way.

When Mikko was 3 years old, I became pregnant with his little brother. My husband Sam and I had purposely spaced out the pregnancies so that Mikko would be able to continue having the *nummies* he loved and needed so strongly. When my milk dried up 10 weeks into the pregnancy, I worried that it would spark a premature and sorrowful weaning, but no, Mikko remained steadfast and dry-nursed throughout the pregnancy.

This, however, was not without its difficulties for me. I was happy that Mikko was still able to derive comfort from nursing, but it was not at all comfortable for my pregnant self. If my pregnancy with him had introduced me to the concept of sore breasts (you know, where even the seat belt in the car and the spray of the shower provoked an *"Ouch!"*), my pregnancy with a toddler dry nursing on said breasts familiarized me with a whole new level of pain. It felt like tiny knives stabbing through my nipples.

I breathed deeply and practiced my childbirth hypnosis techniques. I also began limiting. I started putting Mikko off when he'd want to nurse during the day. With his father's help, I began the task of night weaning him so that I could stay comfortable and get some sleep (a task that was growing more difficult by the month in any case). I explained that my nummies were sore and began cutting short the duration of his nursing sessions. I also insisted on nursing manners: that he sit sedately and in a good position (no toddler acrobatics!) and that he open his mouth wide to latch. It was a compromise for both of us, but it allowed us to make it through the pregnancy with our nursing relationship intact.

At the time, I was mightily relieved. His little brother, Alrik, was born two weeks before Mikko turned 4, and with Mikko's assistance, my milk poured back in the second day postpartum. We were all feeling a little giddy. There was more than enough milk for both of them plus some for me to pump and donate.

Mikko's cheeks plumped up in those first weeks, and this was a testament to the extra calories that he was now once again taking in. He seemed happy to share his nummies with his baby brother, and I was glad to see the tandem breastfeeding smoothing over this huge transition from only child to sibling. Mikko's latch corrected as he relearned how to make the milk flow.

This was all well and good, but...ah, but. I had never before felt nursing aversion and hadn't been expecting it. It hit me hard whenever Mikko nursed. If nails on a chalkboard were a sensation, this would be it. My skin crawled. My sphincters clenched. My teeth ground together. It was all I could do not to toss my dear child, my lovely firstborn preschooler, off my lap and maybe across the room.

I couldn't believe how hard this was. After three easygoing years of breastfeeding and then the unwelcome but expected pain of nursing through pregnancy, I'd thought that getting my milk back would be all that I needed to ensure a simple continuation into tandem nursing and child-led weaning for my older son, but here our paths were diverging. I was feeling more and more strongly that something had to give, that our nursing relationship would need to end for my own mental well-being and the health of our mother–son relationship. Mikko, on the other hand, was blithely continuing to enjoy the renewed milk and the all-day access to the nummies since they were out for his little brother in any case.

I'd been resistant to the idea of mother-led weaning because it didn't jibe with my ideals. I hadn't judged other parents for choosing that route, but I knew that I'd wanted my children's cessation of breastfeeding to be natural and organic.

It took a lot of thought and not a little grieving to realize that I was going to choose mother-led weaning after all. After I'd admitted that fact to myself—the first big hurdle—I could move on to determining how to do it in a way that was as gentle and respectful as possible for Mikko.

The first step was reverting to the techniques that we'd already honed together during the recent pregnancy. I stopped offering the opportunity to breastfeed, and I began to limit the duration and frequency when Mikko requested. We'd developed a signal where I'd say, *"Okay,"* and pat his leg, and he knew it was time then to unlatch and come off. Fortunately for my need to have control over the aversion, he was receptive to this signal, so I knew that I could stop the session if my aversion grew too strong.

Another element that I worked on was dealing with the aversion itself. I didn't want our last nursing sessions to be marred by the heebie-jeebies. I wanted to remember the easy, loving nature of our breastfeeding relationship up until this point, to look down into my first child's babyish face and be flooded instead with the great love that I had for him. I began hypnosis and relaxation techniques again and added to them some mental statements developed by author Amy Phoenix. The one that helped me the most was, *"I choose to breastfeed."* It was so simple yet empowering to realize that it wasn't Mikko causing the aversion or forcing me to experience it. I was in control of my own choice to breastfeed him, and I was bigger than the aversion. I could be a mother to my young son even as I protected my own inner self. This helped me remind myself that I was not a martyr for continuing to breastfeed through pregnancy and now aversion. It was a conscious choice as I prepared for a nurturing end to our breastfeeding relationship. I knew that weaning would still be bittersweet, but I was hoping for less bitter and more sweet.

I realized early on that breastfeeding both children simultaneously was too much stimulation for me, so I began to nurse Mikko only out of Alrik's sight, so he wouldn't scoot over to latch on with his big brother. I reinstituted Mikko's night weaning as well.

Within a few months of his fifth birthday, we were down to two sessions a day: one in the morning after waking up and one in the night before bed. These were both short sessions, sometimes because I stopped him but usually under his own volition. It was clear that he didn't seem to need the feeding aspect of breastfeeding as much anymore. It was more about his checking in for the comfort and security and maybe just the routine. Occasionally, he would ask for nummies at a different time, and I would just tell him we had nummies only in the morning and at night, and he would leave it at that.

Sam and I began talking with him about weaning as well. We pointed out the people in our lives who no longer have nummies from their mamas: his own parents, his beloved cousin, his grandparents and aunts and uncles, and the many friends around his age who'd already weaned. We discussed when he might stop having nummies: maybe at age 5, we suggested? He countered with 7. I suspected that it would be closer to our guess.

I liked that even though my weaning plan was mother-led, it followed a pattern seen in child-led weaning as well: a gradual reduction in nursing frequency and session duration with distractions during the day and deep sleep during the night.

Sure enough, within a few months after his fifth birthday, I realized that Mikko had weaned. He had here and there forgotten to ask for a nursing session, or we'd distracted him in the morning and at night by having his father get him up or put him to bed. I wasn't sure when our absolute last nursing session had been, only that it had been awhile.

I felt—I still feel—wistful about it, but I was also relieved that we'd managed such a peaceful ending when I considered how challenging the final two years of our nursing relationship had been for me. From time to time over the next year, Mikko would hint that he'd still love some nummies, and I would smile at him and say something like, *"Yes, they were very good, weren't they?"* and we'd move on to another topic.

Now at 6, he has finally changed it to the past tense and will sometimes reminisce with me, *"Remember how much I used to love nummies, Mama?"*

Yes, love. Yes, I do.

Not Quite Done After All
Colette Van Heerden, Kwa Zulu Natal, South Africa

B reastfeeding was a definite for me. I had suffered dreadful thrush in my nipples after the birth of my first daughter and ended up weaning her cold turkey at 2 weeks so that my boobs and their open sores could heal. It took me weeks to heal. For two weeks, I did not feed her at all. This was followed by four weeks of slowly reteaching her to breastfeed and supplementing until we were 100% back on *"boob only."*

I fed my first daughter for two years exactly, and we loved it. She was my *"booby baby"* and was not interested in solid food for ages. Breastfeeding for me had been hard in the beginning, but it was 100% worth it. I am so happy when I have a little person tucked into my arms who is safe, warm, and feeling loved.

On the subject of weaning, with my first daughter, I was torn between weaning cold turkey and self-weaning. I went with weaning cold turkey and used bitter aloe on my nipples. The reason was a complete lack of sleep on my part because my daughter was a non-sleeper and woke nine plus times a night! Sleep deprivation was affecting me big time. I thought that if I took breastfeeding out of the equation, I could get her to sleep better and get some sleep myself, and it worked.

After the birth of my second daughter, I contracted shingles and was ignorantly advised by the doctor to not feed my baby because of the meds, so for the second time in my life, I had to stop breastfeeding a brand new little person of mine. She was weaned at 5 days old. After eight days and many tears, I successfully relatched my daughter and continued to exclusively breastfeed her for ages. I knew that I could do it. I'd done it before. I was born to breastfeed.

When my second daughter was 2 years 5 months old, I started going back to the gym. I assumed that my milk supply would dwindle to nothing, and I wrote the following in my daughter's book:

> *"Shortly you will have weaned yourself from my breast. I was always committed to giving you 2 years of breastfeeding, and so very easily, those 2 years came and went. Now, as you stand at 29 months, I can see and feel how natural, right, and easy it has been for us to just carry on together. I knew with you that I wasn't going to do a "cold turkey" to bring breastfeeding to an end. I didn't need to. Our breastfeeding relationship has been an easy one. I was made to breastfeed! I love it! I love that it is nutritious nurturance. I love that it is easy and convenient. I love that it grows you in so many different ways. The way we look into each other's eyes when you feed makes me love, feel in love, feel loved, helps me be loving, and know love. My satisfaction comes from knowing how your touch and my boobs, your suckling and my holding arms can almost cure all and any of your woes and wobbles. We fill each other up when you feed.*
>
> *Now, of course, not every feed is a dream, though most are because, of course, there have been times when I've gotten annoyed that you want boob when I'm busy with work or needing to cook supper. There've been times when at night, all I've wanted you to do is*

sleep—not feed—so that I can sleep too. There are times you struggle to drink when your nose is all stuffy and blocked. However, all of those not-so-fun feeds are but a drop in the ocean. I have tears in my eyes as I write these words, knowing that not only will you miss breastfeeding but that I will too! It is the one act as a mother that really makes me feel like a mom. I hold you close in my arms, your little body snuggled into mine, your wet little mouth, holding my nipple safely within it. Beauty. Innocence. Perfection. Nurturance. Joy. Love."

I did not lose my milk supply, nor did I lose my biggest fan of my ability to breastfeed, my daughter! We just kept right on at it.

Then, when she was nearing 3 years of age, I went through a time of feeling like the tail was wagging the dog. I felt that she had moved through her needing boob to her *"having"* me. Before, she had needed me and breastfeeding to comfort her when she was ill, sore, or tired. Now, it felt like she could get me to jump at her command. I wasn't over the moon with this feeling, but I applied adult thought to it and decided to honor the fact that she was about to be 3 and that it must be her way of showing me that she was now needing to exert some more definite independence of self. So, I embraced it by weaning her after her third birthday.

Not once did I ask if I was ready. Not once did I question whether I felt this was the right thing to do. I thought my way through it, and knowing that I had weaned with aloe before, I chose to do it again.

It was heartache! I cried and cried—big tears, lots of them.

Although I had prepared her and used aloe on my nipples, she responded to my boobs by saying, *"Sgustim"* (disgusting). My experience with her sister was that it was *"done and dusted."* My older daughter never looked back or asked for boob again. My youngest, however, often asked me for boob and then backed away as they got too close. To process the pain that I was going through, I even drew a picture of us breastfeeding together. It was soothing.

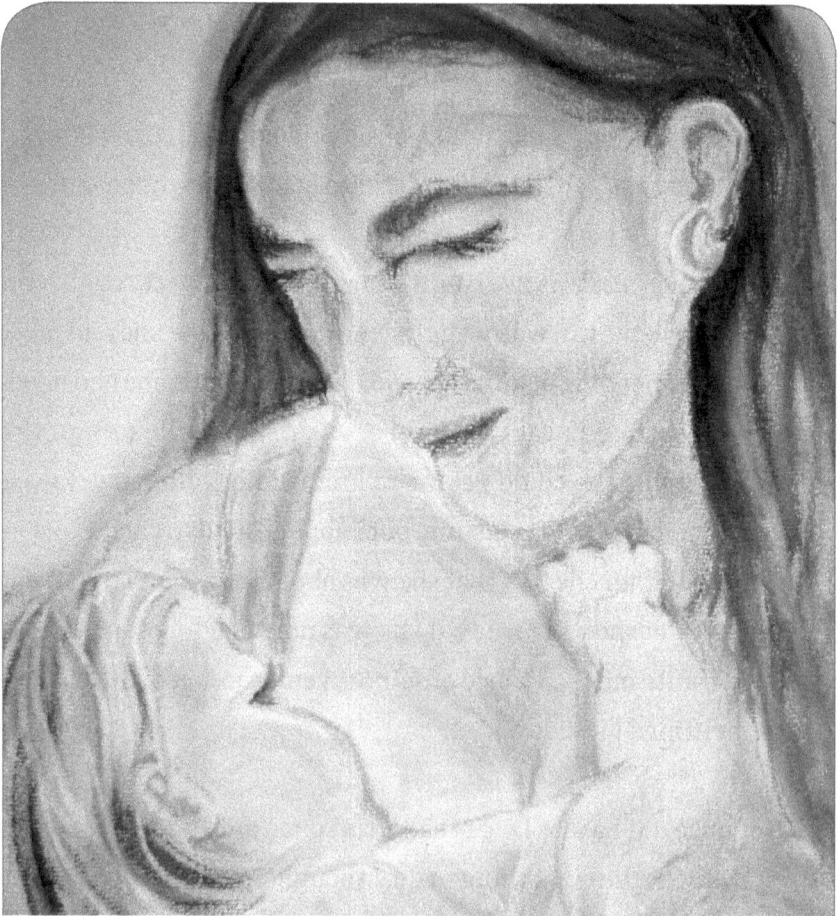

Nutritional nurturance and healing.
Drawn by Colette Van Heerden.

On sharing my misery with a friend, she flippantly suggested that I put honey on my nipples and relatch my little girl that way. So, that night, as my daughter tried again to nestle into my boobs, I gave her my honey-coated nipples, and voila! We were feeding again. Thank you, honey! So, for the second time with my younger daughter, I was successful at relatching her. I was thrilled and elated, and it felt right.

Now, as I write this, she is 4 years 4 months old, and we are still breastfeeding. It is only at night and on waking, but it is something that still feeds us both. I feel that for her, it is still something she needs and enjoys. It has also proved invaluable during those times of illness, when her chest gets her down and my chest (my boobs) still brings her comfort when she is not feeling comfortable herself.

Breastfeeding is our time together for a while longer.

Finding the Right Time to Wean[13]
Heather Holm, Mahone Bay, Nova Scotia

My son almost weaned himself when he was 2 years old. One morning, he declined to nurse when we woke up. I was surprised, but he gave me a hug and said, *"I love you, too."* I didn't feel ready to stop, but I was torn.

On the one hand, I was looking forward to eating what I wanted. My son had food sensitivities that kept him from sleeping well. One small serving for me of a forbidden food could result in a sleepless night two days later after it worked its way through my body into my milk and then into his intestines. We both had to avoid dairy products, gluten, caffeine, chocolate, and hot peppers, all foods I would otherwise eat, just to get a half-decent night's sleep. To fill the nutritional gaps, I was consuming soy products, which weren't so good for me.

On the other hand, I felt sad about weaning. For one thing, with all of the foods that he had to avoid, breast milk was providing him with important nutrition.

Even more importantly, nursing was the one best thing that only I could do to make up for his rough C-section birth. It offered reassurance that the world was safe and okay, reassurance that I felt he still needed. Our close nursing relationship was helping him build a strong, grounded personality so that he could one day face life on his own terms. I realized that I could probably influence him one

---

way or the other but also wanted to respect his wishes. I wanted to do the right thing for him, but what was it?

The next morning when we woke up, he said that he didn't want to nurse. As I rose to get dressed, he saw my breasts and said, *"I nursed them,"* carefully using the past tense, but seeing them made him want to touch them. Touching them made him want to taste them. Tasting them led to a full-blown nursing session. I felt a little guilty that I had tempted him out of his resolve. However, he nursed enthusiastically for another year, and I was glad.

By the time his third birthday came around, I was feeling ready to stop nursing, but he was still enjoying it. At 3 years 2 months old, he was down to taking one breast at a time about twice a day. I weighed the factors and decided that there could be a net benefit to him if we stopped completely at that point.

One fine September afternoon, we were out on the deck nursing. I tried to explain to him how it would be easier to figure out his food sensitivities if he were not getting everything that I had eaten with a day's delay in addition to everything he had eaten himself. He seemed to understand that it was a problem, at least for me.

"I think I could give up nursing," he said generously.

I was surprised, grateful, and a bit apprehensive. *"Okay, then,"* I responded, *"let this be our last nurse."*

The first thing he said the next morning was not, *"I want to nurse,"* as usual, but rather, *"I think I don't want to give up nursing."*

"No, we're not going to nurse anymore," I replied.

He peed in his diaper instead.

Later that day, we got a phone call from an uncle who knew all about breaking a drinking habit. I explained that we were weaning and that his nephew was finding it hard. He promised to send my son a gift when he had been *"dry"* for one month.

On the second day, my son invented a new game in which I was the mother cat and he the kitten. He wanted me to pat him on the head and back like a kitten, rub him behind the ears, pretend to lick him, and be close and snuggly. We would meow and purr for an hour at a time and enjoy playful cuddling without actually nursing.

On the third day, we went sailing. By this time, my breasts were heavy with milk and leaking. I decided that I would have my son empty them at an unexpected time so that it wouldn't remind him too much of old habits. The opportunity came when we dropped anchor at an island. My husband ferried my son and me to the beach to explore and then returned to the sailboat. Eventually my son got hungry, and I had no food with me except what was in my breasts.

"Would you like to nurse one last time?" I asked.

Of course he did, so I sat on a log on the sunny beach, and he had quite a meal. We both felt better in the moment, but there were tears too as I said my final goodbye to breastfeeding.

Over the next few days, he would ask sometimes if my breasts had milk in them.

"We don't do that anymore."

"But I don't want to give up nursing!"

Remembering our experience of the previous year, I didn't dare let him see my breasts during that period.

He started calling me by my first name. *"Why?"* I asked.

"When I was a little baby, I called you Mommy."

A week later, he had stopped asking to nurse in the morning. He might ask once during the day, but I would casually brush it off. He didn't whine about it anymore, but every day he asked, *"What did Uncle say?"*

I would remind him that when he had not nursed for one month, Uncle would send him a gift. *"What is it?"* he wondered, and I had no answer, but thinking about it made him forget about wanting to nurse. A set of plastic dinosaurs soon arrived in the mail, and that sealed the deal.

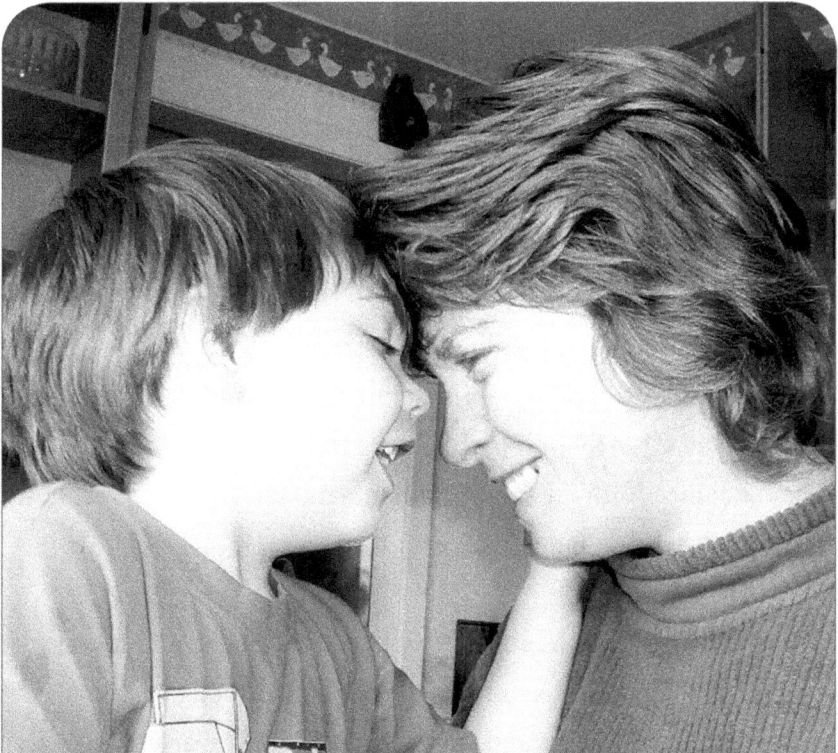

Heather and her son. Photo by Dennis Robinson.

After the miracle of my 42-year-old body making milk for the first time followed by three years of constant production, it seemed amazing that lactation would ever stop. I drank sage tea a couple of times to suppress milk production. However, I think that my milk factories had received the message that demand had dried up, and therefore, the supply line should cease operation. After a week, I was sure that my breasts were no longer filling up, so it was safe for me to eat whatever I wanted: coffee, chocolate, and cheese never tasted so good!

A few weeks after my son's weaning, I noted mental changes in both of us. I was more interested in the news. I could better handle detailed technical issues. I was thinking more about my direction in life. I also observed that my son was expressing a little more aggression. We were now emerging from a cocoon of contentment that had been created by the hormones of lactation.

The day before my next menstrual period, I felt detached and sad. I just wanted to be alone and cry. This short-term depression returned before each period, lessening each month until it was hardly noticeable after five cycles. I'm sure that it was my body finding a new balance without the nursing hormones, just as it would do a few years later at menopause.

Now, I am the mother of a remarkable, confident, and self-assured teenaged boy who has outgrown most of his food sensitivities. I'm sure that our closeness and mutual understanding, grounded in those years of breastfeeding, are making the moods of adolescence easier on both of us. His empathy for me is a reminder that nursing and weaning are carried out as a partnership of two people. We came to know and trust each other as individuals in an intimate setting, and that bond will always be there, even though he consciously remembers little of how it came to be.

There have been other kinds of weaning as we have danced the dance of holding on and letting go that is parenting. Whether it was starting school or flying far away without his parents to visit relatives for a month, each weaning adventure has presented its challenges and its victories for one or both of us. With every step that he takes toward finding his place in the world, it is still my job to provide the security and reassurance that he needs while encouraging the independence that he is ready for.

Weaning from the breast is but one step in the continuum of nurturing and weaning a child.

Weaning at Age 6...Three Times!
Robyn Roche-Paull, RN, IBCLC, Virginia Beach, Virginia[14]

My weaning story actually begins when I was at my six week postpartum visit with my first baby, Morgan. I attended a La Leche League (LLL) meeting on the advice of a nurse at Portsmouth Naval Hospital, who had just attended a weekend course on providing lactation help. At the time, I was on active duty and didn't know where to turn for help with breastfeeding while in the military. The nurse was kindhearted and said that she really didn't know who could help me, but she had heard that LLL was a good resource.

So, off I went to the meeting, which was held in a church resource room. The women were all gathered together, sitting in a circle of chairs with babies in arms and toddlers milling about. The meeting started with the now familiar statement, *"You may see or hear things tonight that are unfamiliar or new to you. We ask that you take what you need and leave the rest."* Boy, was that an understatement! Not 10 minutes into the meeting, the Leader's young son, about 2 years old at the time, climbed up into her lap and calmly lifted her shirt and began to nurse. To say I was dumbfounded is an understatement! I was floored but also very curious. I had never seen a child that age breastfeeding. I have no sisters and only an older brother, and my aunt had breastfed but very discreetly, usually in a bedroom. So, I really didn't have any preconceived notions as to whether it was right or wrong. I do remember thinking that the little toddler seemed so contented and happy but so big on his mother's lap! I looked down at my little 6-week-old baby boy and wondered briefly if he would ever be that big, and I thought that if I managed to breastfeed for six months, much less two years, it was going to be a miracle! Little did I know what was in store for me.

Fast forward through the first year of his life, when I worked 12- to 18-hour days as an aircraft mechanic in the U.S. Navy. I pumped every 2 to 3 hours while I was at work and coslept and breastfed on demand while I was at home. I dealt with hazardous material exposure, unsupportive coworkers and supervisors, and a flight schedule that often left me with full, aching breasts and bouts of mastitis when I had no time to pump.

Somehow, my little boy and I persevered, and his first birthday came and went with no sign of him wanting to wean. I wasn't in any hurry either since I didn't have to pump anymore for work and could just enjoy coming home after work to a hungry boy who wanted nothing more than his *"munyas,"* his word for breastfeeding, and a snuggle with me. His second birthday also came and went, and again, I saw no reason to wean him. We were both enjoying our breastfeeding relationship too much to quit, and besides, he still looked so little to me. I was his rock, his base to come back to as he explored the world around him. His dad, who was also on active duty in the U.S. Navy, was gone on deployment that year, and we both missed him a lot. Breastfeeding helped to soothe both our souls until he returned.

With my husband's return from deployment, I found myself pregnant—big surprise, right?—and in uncharted waters. My eldest showed no signs of weaning, and my nipples were incredibly sore.

Once again, my LLL group saved the day, as I was able to get information and support for continuing to breastfeed through the pregnancy and for tandem nursing after my daughter was born. Now that my son could talk, he would tell me that my milk tasted funny and that it was very hard to get out, but that he really, really needed to have his munyas, so he was not going to stop, and he didn't. He nursed throughout the pregnancy. Oftentimes, I had to count to 20 or go through the alphabet, and he knew to stop when I got to the end. I nursed him right up to my labor with her.

After she was born, he latched right back on and shared his first tandem-nursing session with her when she was a mere 20 minutes old. In the coming days, my milk came in. His face lit up, and he told me, *"Mommy, the munyas are back!"* Oh, happy days! He nursed like never before, put on baby fat again, and acted like a milk-drunk fool for a few days. My daughter, Siobhan, nursed right alongside him, and they often held hands together in the first year. In her second and third years of life, they both continued to tandem-nurse together but with far more fighting then handholding. My lap was shrinking, what with one toddler and one preschooler both breastfeeding at the same time!

By this time, I felt like a pro regarding breastfeeding an older child. My eldest was down to nursing just in the mornings and before bed. We could carry on conversations about breastfeeding, why he liked it, what it tasted like, and so on. My daughter would chime in with her thoughts too, which often led to more arguments about the supposed flavor of milk from each breast or which side was better. My son was going to enter kindergarten in the fall, and I didn't know anyone who had breastfed a kindergartner! I figured that it would work itself out and that he would quit when he was ready. I didn't have long to wait.

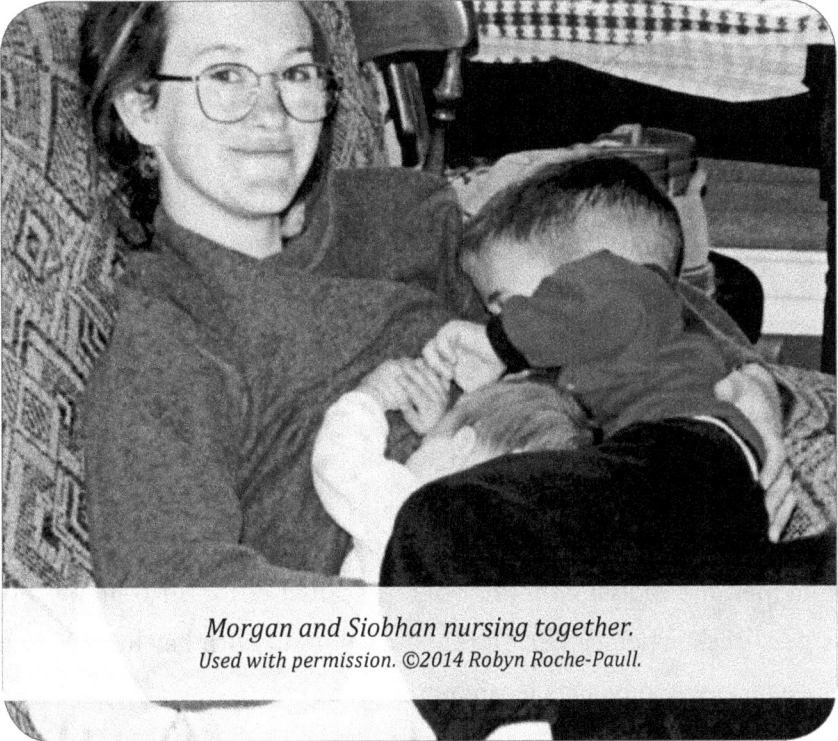

Morgan and Siobhan nursing together.
Used with permission. ©2014 Robyn Roche-Paull.

After a year of trying for our third baby, I finally got pregnant. However, I didn't find out by the usual means of a pregnancy test. While I was nursing my then 6-year-old son, he pulled away and said that my milk tasted horrible and that it reminded him of when I was pregnant with his sister. I did some quick calculations in my head and realized that he was right. My period was late, and it was the right timing for me to be pregnant. I took a pregnancy test later that day, and it was positive. He weaned the next morning at the age of 6½ years and told me that he loved the munyas but could not stand to deal with the bad taste again, and that he didn't need it anymore like he did when he was little. That was that: no muss and no fuss. He weaned when he was ready and told me that I was pregnant with his brother!

My daughter continued to nurse throughout the pregnancy without batting an eye. She never complained about the taste changing or my supply going down. She was always a much more efficient and quick breastfeeder and only nursed long enough to satisfy her needs. Then, she was off and running, unlike her brother, who would linger and dillydally. However, I had to do the same with her and count to 10 or 20 or go through the alphabet when the nipple soreness or *"twitchy"* feelings got to be too much.

Soon enough, I was at the end of the pregnancy and in labor with her little brother. She actually nursed throughout my labor and helped me to kick-start it when it stalled out after 6 hours. Like her brother before her, she tandem-nursed with her little brother Tiernan when he was fresh out of the womb.

Two years passed with Siobhan and Tiernan tandem-nursing together, with the usual amounts of handholding interspersed with fighting and arguing over who had which side last. When my daughter was approaching her sixth birthday, I wondered if she would continue or if the end was nearing for her as well. I shouldn't have been surprised that the little girl who wouldn't stay on the breast for more than 10 minutes at a time would be the one to state that she was weaning on her sixth birthday and then do it. She woke up that morning and stated she was done with having *"nanas"* and ran off to play. She never looked back and never again asked to breastfeed after that day.

Once again, weaning was so easy. It just happened when the time was right, and there were no tears or worries on the part of me or my daughter. My youngest continued to nurse after his sister weaned. At first, he was thrilled to have the *"nummies"* all to himself, but gradually, I began to see that he was nursing less and less. I think that because there was not another child to keep the milk supply up, I was drying up more quickly than before. I wondered if he would make it to 6 years or not.

Early in his sixth year, we were interviewed for a *20/20* special on extended breastfeeding, and the reporter asked Tiernan how long he was going to nurse. He stated that he would nurse until he was 9 years old because it was good and made him feel happy. That was a bittersweet moment for me as I sensed the end was near. He was nursing less and less by that point, skipping days and sometimes going a whole week without nursing. Shortly after the TV show, he weaned when his grandparents invited him to go on a trip. He and I talked about how I wouldn't be there for him to have his nummies, but he said that it was okay. He was a big boy now and had been looking forward to finally going on a trip with his Nanu and Bampa (like his older siblings had been doing after they weaned). He left for the week-long Easter break trip, and when he came back, he never asked to nurse again.

That was it. The end of 13 straight years of breastfeeding came to a close. I felt both relieved and sad. I was relieved to have my breasts back and to not have someone touching them, sucking on them, fondling them, and generally just being on them all the time, but I was sad to see the end of an era that had brought my children and I such happiness, such intimacy, such closeness. I knew that I would never have those moments again.

My children have continued to remain close and are willing to talk to me about anything and everything and have snuggles on the couch while we are watching a movie, even as they have become teenagers. However, I still occasionally miss those wonderfully close moments that one feels only when there is a child at the breast. I look back at that LLL meeting where I saw a toddler breastfeeding for the first time and laugh at myself. I had no idea what I was getting into that day, but I am so glad that I went to that meeting and kept an open mind about it all. I am proud that I breastfed my three children to the age of 6 years and that they each weaned when they were ready and not a moment before. I am so glad that I could give that gift to them.

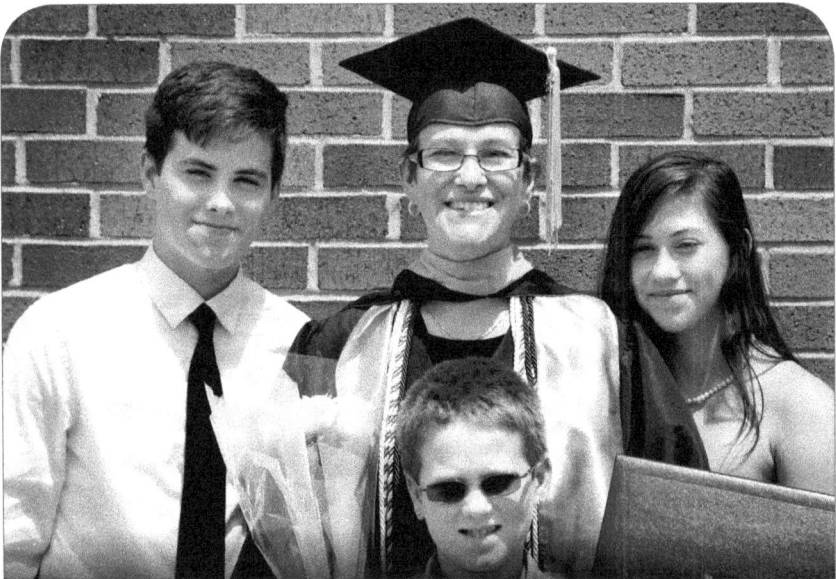

Morgan, Tiernan, Robyn, and Siobhan at Robyn's graduation from nursing school. Used with permission. ©2014 Robyn Roche-Paull.

Postscript by Siobhan Paull

My name is Siobhan (pronounced Shavon), and my mother is Robyn. I'm 15 years old, and I nursed until I was 6 years old. What I mostly remember about nursing is that I enjoyed it. It gave me a protective feeling, being in my mom's lap and having that skin-to-skin contact. Also knowing that she was there holding me gave me that feeling of love and care.

One of the positive effects that breastfeeding had on me when I was growing up was the relationship with my mom. I think that if I hadn't been breastfed, I wouldn't be as open with her and be as willing to confide stuff to her. I can't really think of any negative effect that breastfeeding had on my mother or myself.

I nursed for six years, and some people would say that is a long time, but the truth is that I weaned myself. There was no pressure from my mom at all. I just said one night, *"I want to quit on my sixth birthday,"* and I went to bed like a big girl. When I woke up the next morning, I stopped cold turkey.

I think that nursing for six years had an effect on me being independent, just not that big of an effect. I don't think that it was breastfeeding that made me independent. It's the fact that breastfeeding gave me that special bond with my momma, which gave me independence. One thing that I did when I was breastfeeding that I don't mind sharing is that when I would breastfeed, I would always comment on the flavor. It would either be orange in the right breast and chocolate in the left or vice versa, and sometimes, the chocolate would be vanilla. I think that this shows my sense of humor when I was little.

Morning Cuddles
Janell E. Robisch, Luray, Virginia

Although I couldn't see it at the time, my firstborn's weaning was a constant back-and-forth balancing of needs that eventually came to a peaceful end. It was tied in with his need to be close to me and to continue to nurse and my need to reduce the feeling of being touched out and my fear of not being able to conceive again until he was done nursing.

Whether it is scientifically proven or not, I believe that a mother's body and mind have a special way of knowing what is best for the child that she has and that nursing only strengthens that bond and that knowledge. I wouldn't be surprised if they someday find special hormonal or pheremonal connections between nursing and fertility. It's the only way that I can explain how my body's fertility changed so drastically between the births of each of my children.

It took me two-and-a-half years of trying to conceive before my first child, A.J., was born. He was a superintelligent and high-needs child, but since he was my only one, after our initial getting-used-to-being-parents stage, life with him was very doable and enjoyable. I had many the *"A-ha"* moment about his needs and behavior later on when he was diagnosed with Asperger's syndrome and anxiety issues at age 8.

I conceived once more before the end of his nursing, ironically when he had gone a week or so without *"nursies,"* but that pregnancy sadly ended in a miscarriage at nine weeks. When I conceived again, only three months later, A.J. was done with nursing altogether. He ended up being six years older than his first sister, Lily. The big shocker fertility-wise came when I got pregnant with my second daughter, Ginny, when Lily was only 12 months old and still going strong when it came to milk. It would be another four years before Lily weaned, so she was nowhere close to being done at this stage.

When A.J. was still nursing, I often entertained the idea that my body couldn't get pregnant again until he weaned. I got my period back when he was 10 months old, but I still couldn't get pregnant. For some reason, I felt that he needed me that much, and somehow, through nursing and constant contact, my body knew it.

I didn't resent him for this, however. The two-and-a-half years that it took for me to conceive him in the first place made me appreciate the fact that I might never have another child. I quickly decided to act in favor of the child I had versus the child I might one day have.

That's not to say that I didn't cry about the situation or bemoan my inability to conceive another child occasionally, but I never blamed my sweet boy for the situation.

So, when I was feeling touched out or just ready to quit nursing, I would test the waters, cut back a little, or talk to A.J. about it and see how he reacted. I felt that since I was the adult, I could be patient when I needed to. If his reaction was intense, I knew that he wasn't ready, like the many short-lived occasions when I tried night weaning. If, however, he went on about his business without much reaction to what I was doing—or not doing—I knew that we could move forward.

The following excerpt from my personal journal, written in 2006, tells the rest of the story:

"When my son finally weaned in January 2006 at age 5 years 3 months, of course, part of me wondered if I had done the right thing in nudging him along. I had been ready to end nursing for a while but was contented to let him continue to nurse until he was really ready to stop. To me, 'ready to stop' meant that he would not be traumatized by weaning and that, as a mother and child, we would be able to easily meet his needs in other ways.

About four months before he actually weaned, A.J. set a date for weaning. During the interval before that date, he continued to nurse in the same pattern, in the morning and before bed and sometimes in between. However, when the date actually came, he said that he was going to stop nursing for that day only. I smiled and waited a while longer to bring up the subject again. About a month later, he stopped nursing for six days but then went back to it.

It was the end of November when we talked about it again. He had just turned 5 in October. I suggested that it might be easier for him if he got used to the idea of weaning by slowing down a little at a time. He was amenable to the idea and set yet another date. This time, however, he did slow his nursing down right away; he suddenly went days without any nursies and showed no ill effects. In addition, prospects for a weaning party were suddenly more important than having milk.

The last day of nursies (January 1) came and went, and we even took pictures of his last nurse. As things went, he came down with a stomach bug a few weeks later, and he did nurse one more time around January 18.

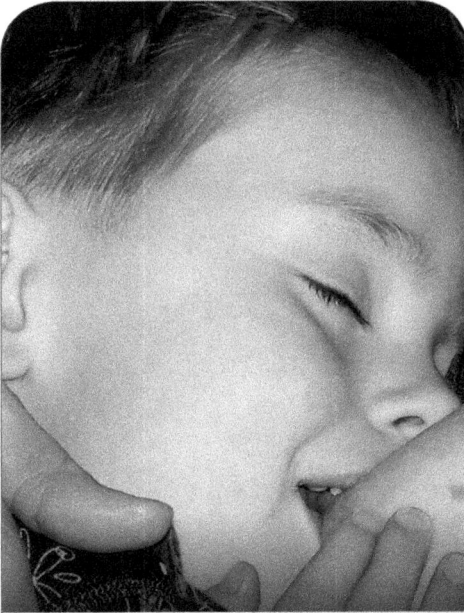

A.J. saying a cheerful
and tender goodbye to nursies.
©2006 Janell E. Robisch.

Now, as I write this, five months later in May 2006, I am confident that we did okay. He has not asked to nurse again since that day and has not shown any ill effects of weaning. We still have plenty of close cuddle time, especially every morning when he wakes up. If I am not nearby when he wakes, he seeks me out as he still likes to start his day with some close time with Mommy. Our bond is still there, still strong, even though our nursing relationship is over. I will be ever grateful for the bond that it created and am happy that we had that special time together."

It has been eight years since I wrote that journal entry. A.J. is now 13 years old and is still incredibly smart and exacting. He is not incredibly *"touchy"* with most people, but he always makes time for a hug for me when he first wakes up and before he goes to bed. Our relationship, like any mother–child relationship, is not perfect, but I feel that nursing, more than anything, laid down a foundation of love and connection for us that will last a lifetime.

Appendix A

Milky Names

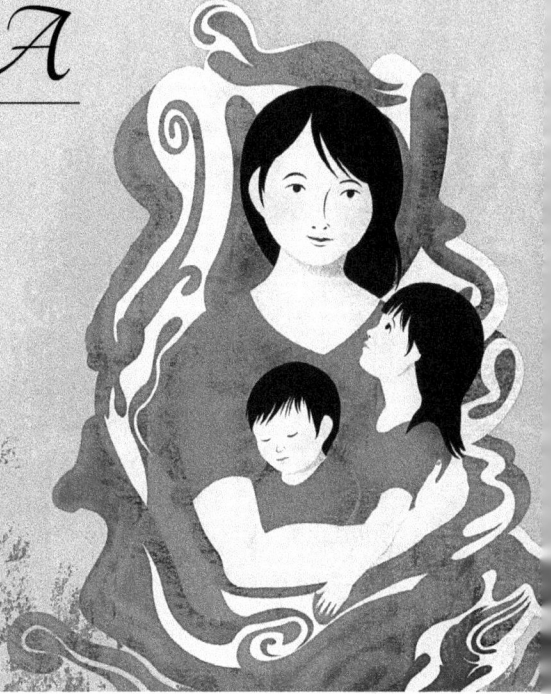

Some names for nursing come about naturally and stem from the way mother and baby talk. Other names are created as less obvious *"code words"* for a nursling to use in public.

Whatever the case, I've collected a variety of sometimes amusing names that mothers and children that I've known and talked to use for the one and only breast milk.

Aside

Ba

Baba

Baby

Big Fat Sideydidey

Boob

Boobie/Boobee/Booby

Boobie Snacks

Booboos

Boosies

Breast

Bub

Che-Che (from the Spanish word leche)

Comida

Cuddles

Cuddling

Dee-Dee ("this side")

Durts

Freshies

Heh-heh

Hop

Hym Hym

I want one./I want the other one.

I want to nurse.

Kitse

Latuzzu (slang for "milkies" in Italian)

M-M or M&M (short for mom's milk)

Ma

Mama

Mama Milk/Mama's Milk

Mama More

Mamas

Mee-Mee Milk Mamma

Mee-Mees/Mimi

Meems

Me-Me Milk

Mexican (mispronunciation of the German Milch trinken)

Milk

Milka/Milkas

Milkie/Milkies/Milky

Milktaplease

Moke

Mommy Milk/Mommy's Milk

Mommy Moo/Pink Momy Moo/ Ummy Pink Mommy Moo

Mommy More

More

Muk

Mum

Mummy Eat

Munyas

NaNa/Na-Na/Na-Nas/Nanas

Nang/Nang Nangs

Nannies/Nanny

Nanno

Nanoo

Nanu Juice

Nee

Neena

Nee-Nee/Ni-Ni

Nee-Nee Now

Nene

Nigh

Nigh Nigh's

Nin

Ninnies

Nippies

Nonie

Noonie/Noonies

Num Nums

Nummies/Nummy

Num-Num/Num-Nums

Nun

Nu-Nu

Nur

Nurse

Nursie/Nursies

Nursing

Onnee

Other

Roun-er-Roun (for turning around
  while nursing)

Side/Sides

Teta

That

Tittymilk

Want to Nurse

Yie (for "side")

Appendix B

International Breastfeeding Resources

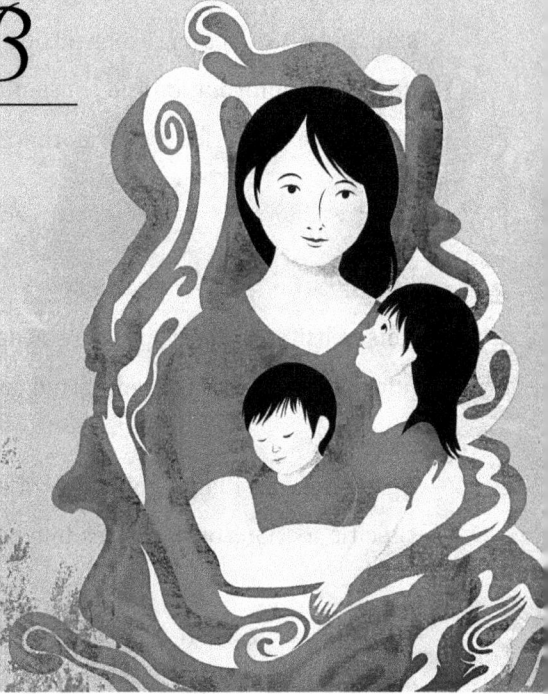

This is a small collection of international breastfeeding resources, all of which have a presence online. You may find helpful articles from the Australian Breastfeeding Association even if you are in the United States or Europe. Through these organizations, you might find helpful information on full-term and extended nursing and access to in-person, online, or telephone breastfeeding counselors or local support groups. I've tried to stick to free or not-for-profit groups that are as accessible as possible.

Australian Breastfeeding Association
http://www.breastfeeding.asn.au/

"The Australian Breastfeeding Association (ABA) is Australia's largest breastfeeding information and support service. Breastfeeding is a practical, learned skill, and ABA helps more than 80,000 mothers each year. ABA also provides up-to-date information and continuing education for thousands of health professionals working with mothers and babies."

KellyMom
http://kellymom.com/category/bf/

"This website was developed to provide evidence-based information on breastfeeding and parenting."

KellyMom has a large collection of articles on breastfeeding, including specific sections on breastfeeding past 1 year and weaning.

La Leche League International
http://www.llli.org

"Our Mission is to help mothers worldwide to breastfeed through mother-to-mother support, encouragement, information, and education, and to promote a better understanding of breastfeeding as an important element in the healthy development of the baby and mother."

La Leche League offers a large collection of informational articles on its website as well as access to its vast networks of local volunteer La Leche League Leaders, who provide one-on-one breastfeeding support, and local groups all over the world.

The Breastfeeding Network (United Kingdom)
http://www.breastfeedingnetwork.org.uk/

"The Breastfeeding Network (BfN) aims to be an independent source of support and information for breastfeeding women and others...The Breastfeeding Network is a recognised Scottish Charity (SC027007)....It aims to:

» promote breastfeeding and a greater understanding of breastfeeding in the United Kingdom.

» collect and disseminate information on breastfeeding and baby and infant nutrition.

» provide information and support to parents on the feeding of babies and infants.

» set and encourage the acceptance of quality standards for breastfeeding support.

» establish and publish codes of practice for such support."

To Three and Beyond Facebook Community
https://www.facebook.com/groups/660759677271153/

This group is for the support and discussion of breastfeeding to the third birthday and beyond and of the book *To Three and Beyond.* Approval of the list owner/moderator is required to join. The group's privacy settings are closed, which means that anyone can see the group and who is in it, but only members can see posts.

Womenshealth.gov
http://www.womenshealth.gov/breastfeeding/

"The experience of breastfeeding is special for so many reasons—the joyful bonding with your baby, the cost savings, and the health benefits for both mother and baby. Read on for tips and suggestions to help you successfully breastfeed."

World Alliance for Breastfeeding Action (WABA)
http://www.waba.org.my/

"WABA is a global network of organizations and individuals who believe breastfeeding is the right of all children and mothers, and who dedicate themselves to protect, promote, and support this right. WABA acts on the Innocenti Declaration and works in close liaison with UNICEF."

WABA also publishes a mother support newsletter, which is available at http://www.waba.org.my/whatwedo/gims/index.htm.

Appendix C

What Science Has to Say

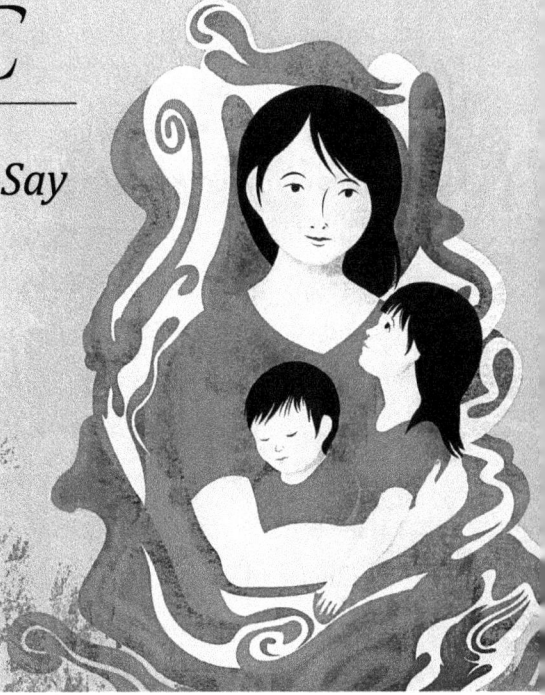

Although this book is mainly about the personal experiences of mothers who choose to breastfeed their children past their third birthdays, I feel that it is necessary to back up these choices a bit with some information from scientific research from anthropological, social, and biological perspectives.

With a viewpoint stemming from the 20th-century use of formula, many opponents of long-term nursing seem to see breastfeeding past a year or so as unnatural. Children in our society are frequently expected to be independent from a very early age—to sleep through the night by 6 weeks and to follow a strict schedule of meeting what can seem like arbitrary milestones. Any variation from this preformed schedule, which seems to have no respect for the needs and abilities of individual children, causes parents and health care providers to become nervous and filled with worry.

A child who is still nursing at age 4 is almost unheard of, but perhaps many mothers are, in a quiet way, following their instincts after all, despite ill-informed comments and advice. Mothers are in a unique position to observe their children's individual personalities and to recognize that their needs may be different from those listed on a chart. However, it takes a lot of confidence to stand up against the norm and to come *"out of the closet"* with a behavior that is perceived by many to be weird at best and sexual or abusive at worst. Each mother without support must constantly reinvent the wheel and figure out what is best for her child, and she may be fighting society's current norms as she does.

In an attempt to provide some support for these mothers in the form of scientific research and inquiry, here I look back at what has been considered natural and normal worldwide throughout history instead of what is considered normal through the narrow lens of our industrialized 21st-century culture.

In a study that is famous in breastfeeding circles, Kathryn Dettwyler[15] attempted to establish a biological *"hominid blueprint"* for

15   (a) Dettwyler, K. A. (1994). A Time to Wean. *Breastfeeding Abstracts*, 14(1), 3–4. Retrieved from https://www.llli.org/ba/aug94.html. (b) *Breastfeeding: Biocultural Perspectives.* (1995). Stuart-Macadam, P., & Dettwyler, K. A., Eds. de Gruyter: New York. (c) Dettwyler, K. A. (1995/1997). *A Natural Age of Weaning.* Retrieved from http://www.whale.to/a/dettwyler.html.

weaning by gathering evidence from nonhuman primates and less industrialized human cultures. She concluded on the basis of primate data that the natural human age for weaning is between 2½ and 7 years.

In addition, even though generally safe foods and medicine are available in our industrialized society, she stated that children who are breastfed still have an edge, both physically and in terms of emotional attachment, over those that are not.[16] She mentioned that *"another important consideration for the older child is that they are able to maintain their emotional attachment to a person, rather than being forced to switch to an inanimate object such as a teddy bear or blanket."*

With a perspective that is perhaps more common to many in industrialized societies, Muriel Sugarman and Kathleen Kendall-Tackett[15] studied the ages and methods of weaning in a sample of women practicing extended breastfeeding. They found that the average age of weaning in their study was between 2 years 6 months and 3 years 0 months, and the overall age of weaning ranged from 1 month to 7 years 4 months. These numbers were more similar to those of mothers in traditional cultures than those of typical North American mothers, and they suggest that mothers in industrialized societies, especially those already committed to breastfeeding for at least a year, may follow practices that are more similar to those in traditional societies but may not be as outward about it for fear of social repercussions.

---

16   Sugarman, M., & Kendall-Tackett, K. A. (1995). Weaning ages in a sample of women who practice extended breastfeeding. *Clinical Pediatrics, 34*, 642–647.

We have all heard of the benefits of breastfeeding. Breastfeeding in general has been shown to have many benefits.

Here is a short review of some of them:

» *In children, "breastfeeding was associated with a reduction in the risk of acute otitis media, non-specific gastroenteritis, severe lower respiratory tract infections, atopic dermatitis, asthma (young children), obesity, type 1 and 2 diabetes, childhood leukemia, sudden infant death syndrome (SIDS), and necrotizing enterocolitis."[17]*

» *Children who were breastfed for longer than six months were shown to be at lower risk for mental health problems in their teen years.[18]*

» *Longer durations of breastfeeding have been shown to have greater effects in several areas. Advantages for breastfed children include protection against obesity and improved cognitive performance. Advantages for breastfeeding mothers include protection against maternal type 2 diabetes and rheumatoid arthritis.[19]*

» *Women who breastfed their children were found to have a lower risk for Alzheimer's disease than women who did not.[20]*

» *Breastfeeding reduces the risks of reproductive cancers, heart disease, and osteoporosis in breastfeeding mothers.[21]*

---

17   Ip, S., Chung, M., Raman, G., Chew, P., Magula, N., Devine, D., Trikalinos, T. and Lau, J. (2007). Breastfeeding and maternal and infant health outcomes in developed countries. *Evidence Reports/Technology Assessments,* No. 153; Report No. 07-E007.

18   Oddy, W. H., Kendall, G. E., Li, J., Jacoby, P., Robinson, M., de Klerk, N. H., Silburn, S. R., Zubrick, S. R., Landau, L. I., & Stanley, F. J. (2010). The long-term effects of breastfeeding on child and adolescent mental health: A pregnancy cohort study followed for 14 years. *Journal of Pediatrics,* 156, 568–574.

19   Harmon-Jones, C. (2006). Duration, intensity, and exclusivity of breastfeeding: Recent research confirms the importance of these variables. *Breastfeeding Abstracts,* 25, 17–20.

20   Fox, M., Berzuini, C., & Knapp, L. A. (2013). Maternal breastfeeding history and Alzheimer's disease risk. *Journal of Alzheimer's Disease Risk,* 37, 809–821.

21   Dermer, A. (2001). A well-kept secret: Breastfeeding's benefits to mothers. *New Beginnings,* 18, 124–127.

Despite these advantages, many mothers who practice long-term breastfeeding have come across someone—a friend, family member, or medical professional—who has contended that breastfeeding past some mysterious age, be it 6 months, 1 year, or 3 years, has no benefits and may be harmful. These people seem to believe that breast milk magically loses its nutritional and immunological value as the baby ages, although there is no evidence to support this theory.

According to the Australian Breastfeeding Association[22]

> *"Breast milk never loses its nutritional and protective value. Breast milk changes to meet the needs of a child. It continues to provide excellent nutrition, immune and other health and emotional benefits for as long as a child continues to breastfeed."*

Ann Prentice,[23] in *Food and Nutrition Bulletin*, stated that:

> *"Breast milk can continue to be a valuable nutrient source and to provide non-nutritional factors even for older children."*

To be fair, however, studies on breastfeeding and the composition of human milk a year or more into lactation are few and far between. This leaves both supporters and opponents of long-term breastfeeding to draw their own conclusions.

---

22   *Breastfeeding: Fact or fiction?* Australian Breastfeeding Association. Retrieved from https://www.breastfeeding.asn.au/bfinfo/breastfeeding-fact-or-fiction.

23   Prentice, A. (1996). Constituents of human milk. *Food & Nutrition Bulletin*, 17(4), 305–312.

Nutrition and immunological benefits are certainly important, and they often start out as the primary reasons for initiating breast-feeding. However, as the child ages, especially in industrialized cultures, these generally seem to become more side benefits, with bonding, comfort, behavior modification, and the child's own wishes becoming the most important reasons that mothers continue to breastfeed their children past toddlerhood.

In the end, it seems that each mother must do what mothers have always done: weigh the advantages and disadvantages of continuing to breastfeed and those of weaning and decide what is best for her and her child.

This is a decision that belongs in the hands of mother and child and should be dictated by their individual needs and not by society's general norms.

Editor's Note

Please note the following clarification from Katherine Dettwyler. Used with permission. http://www.kathydettwyler.org/commentaries/weaning.html

One often hears that the worldwide average age of weaning is 4.2 years, but this figure is neither accurate nor meaningful. A survey of 64 "traditional" studies done prior to the 1940s showed a median duration of breastfeeding of about 2.8 years, but with some societies breastfeeding for much shorter, and some for much longer. It is meaningless, statistically, to speak of an average age of weaning worldwide, as so many children never nurse at all, or their mothers give up in the first few days, or at six weeks when they go back to work. It is true that there are still many societies in the world where children are routinely breastfed until the age of four or five years or older, and even in the United States, some children are nursed for this long and longer. In societies where children are allowed to nurse "as long as they want" they usually self-wean, with no arguments or emotional trauma, between 3 and 4 years of age.

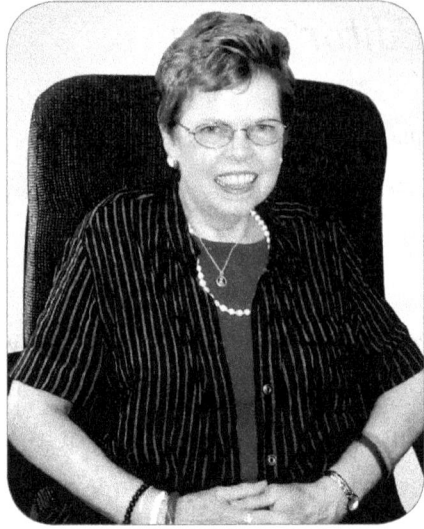

Remembering Judy Torgus

The editors of *Clinical Lactation* were saddened to learn that our colleague and friend, Judy Torgus, passed away quietly in her sleep July 3. Judy was an editor at La Leche League International for over 30 years and served as head of their publications department. Marian Tompson, a founder of La Leche League said that "many of the books published by LLLI came about because of Judy's determination to get needed information into the hands of breastfeeding mothers." After retiring from LLLI, she worked as a freelance editor and assisted me in the production process of *Clinical Lactation* in its earliest days. She also edited books for us at Praeclarus Press. The book, *To Three and Beyond,* a compilation of mothers' stories about toddler nursing, was the last book she edited. That her last book was about mothers' stories seems particularly apt. Both *Clinical Lactation* and Praeclarus Press benefitted from her expertise, her passion for breastfeeding and helping new mothers, and her (at times) wicked sense of humor. I will miss her.

Kathleen Kendall-Tackett, PhD, IBCLC, RLC, FAPA

Editor-in-Chief

www.ingramcontent.com/pod-product-compliance
Lightning Source LLC
Chambersburg PA
CBHW072118270326
41931CB00010B/1596